THE
CHINESE
WAY TO
HEALTH

THE
CHINESE
WAY TO
HEALTH

A Self-help Guide
to Traditional
Chinese Medicine

DR STEPHEN GASCOIGNE

QI GONG CONSULTANT
James MacRitchie

CHINESE MASSAGE CONSULTANT
Robert Cran

PHOTOGRAPHY BY
Gill Orsman

Hodder & Stoughton

To my father, Bill, with love and affection

Text copyright © Dr Stephen Gascoigne 1997
Photographs copyright © Gill Orsman 1997
Photographs copyright © Stephen Marwood 1997
Illustrations copyright © Julie Carpenter 1997
This edition copyright © Eddison Sadd Editions 1997

First published in Great Britain in 1997 by Hodder and Stoughton.
A Division of Hodder Headline Plc.

1 3 5 7 9 10 8 6 4 2

A CIP catalogue record for this book is available from the British Library.

ISBN 0 340 68175 6

AN EDDISON·SADD EDITION
Edited, designed and produced by
Eddison Sadd Editions Limited
St Chad's House, 148 King's Cross Road
London WC1X 9DH

Phototypeset in Venetian 301 BT and Trajan MT using QuarkXPress on Apple Macintosh
Origination by Columbia Overseas Marketing Pte Ltd, Singapore
Printed and bound by Dai Nippon Printing Company (Hong Kong) Ltd

Hodder and Stoughton
A Division of Hodder Headline PLC
338 Euston Road
London NW1 3BH

CONTENTS

INTRODUCTION

Health has been described as our greatest gift – after all, everyone wants to know how to keep in the best state of health and well-being. Western medicine, while excelling at treating life-threatening diseases, traumatic injury and crisis intervention, falls far short of understanding or effectively treating chronic disease and degeneration. This is where Chinese medicine comes into its own. Chinese medicine has a unique view of the whole person as an energetic network of interconnecting channels and organs, and as such it is increasingly being recognized as one of the great resources for promoting health and treating disease.

Today, more and more people are turning to such ancient wisdoms, and there are a number of reasons for this. Some need help with specific health problems, some wish to experience continuing good health and an increased sense of well-being, whilst others have a deep feeling of connection with Chinese or oriental philosophies. Whatever your situation, you will find that Chinese medicine has the breadth of view and the profundity of knowledge to help and support you.

When I worked in conventional medical practice in the late 1970s and early 1980s, there was little mention of Chinese medicine. My first experience of it was when some of my patients returned to me with relief of their symptoms, not from anything that I had done but because they had received acupuncture or herbal treatment. From this point on, I became more and more interested in what Chinese medicine had to offer. I subsequently trained in Chinese medicine and have found it to be extremely effective, safe and gentle. Since then, it seems that almost everyone has heard of acupuncture (one of the main professional treatments), and it is now increasingly common to come across Chinese herbal medicine, *Qi Gong, Tai Chi Chuan*, Chinese massage (*An Mo* and *Tui Na*) and other aspects of the vast treasury that is Chinese medicine. Many people have already had such treatments, and many more are considering receiving them.

WHAT IS CHINESE MEDICINE?

Chinese medicine is a holistic system of medicine which originated in China at least 4,000 years ago. Over the intervening centuries it has spread from its origins and can now be found worldwide. It provides the basic philosophical foundation for related medical systems in neighbouring countries such as Korea, Japan and Vietnam; some practitioners use the term 'oriental medicine' to include these influences.

The underlying principle is that energy – *Qi* (pronounced 'chee') – pervades the whole of the body and the surrounding environment. Health is when the flow of Qi is balanced and harmonious. The philosophical basis of Chinese medicine is that Qi flows because of a constant dynamic process between two poles, *yin* and *yang*. The whole universe can be understood in terms of these two aspects, and, when applied to the individual, they can lead to the treatment of disease. This, essentially, is Chinese medicine; the principles are universal and can be applied to us all. A development of the yin–yang theory – the five elements (*see page 30*) – is of great help in understanding the function of our internal organs and their interaction with nature.

MODERN HEALTH-CARE

In the past twenty years or so, people in the West have started to think differently about health and disease. As people begin to take more responsibility for their health, they are becoming more familiar with systems of healing such as Chinese medicine, which include, rather than exclude, their active participation.

Chinese medicine has always been primarily concerned with maintaining health rather than with merely treating disease and ill-health. It is excellent in dealing with disease when it occurs, but prevention is always preferable to cure. There is a Chinese saying that treating an illness is like digging a well when thirsty. That is to say, there may be some benefit in doing so but preparing before the event is the best policy.

The Chinese, therefore, have a positive view of health and being 'human'. Health is not just the absence of symptoms but the presence of a vital and dynamic state of well-being. You may know from your own experience that there are times when you feel 'under the weather' or below par – you do not have a disease and but there is something not quite right. Chinese medicine can explain – and correct – such feelings. This will help to prevent the development of more serious problems later and also allow you to benefit from increased feelings of vitality.

METHODS OF TREATMENT

The beauty of Chinese medicine is that it gives you a simple yet profound understanding of how the body works and its connections with the environment. By changing our habits or applying specific treatments, it is possible to correct any irregularities and generally to strengthen ourselves as a whole. If the flow of Qi becomes disordered, either due to a weakness in the Qi or because its flow is not smooth, then this can lead to the development of symptoms within the body.

There are eight methods available to Chinese medicine which can be used to prevent or treat illness (*see below*). They are all effective in regaining and supporting health. A variety of approaches is always helpful in any situation as treatment can be tailored to individual needs. A simple adjustment to an aspect of lifestyle may be sufficient – perhaps diet or exercise; if not, more powerful methods such as acupuncture and herbs can be used.

Meditation

This is considered to be the most powerful method for attaining good health. It affects us on every level, helping not just physically, but also psychologically and, ultimately, spiritually. Meditation is discussed in chapter three, along with some simple meditation exercises for you to try.

Food

Many cultures have realized that the type of food eaten, how it is prepared and how it is eaten has a powerful effect on our health. The Chinese, with their insights into Qi and the subtle energetic workings of the body, have set out clearly how various foods affect different organs, and how diet may be changed to counter the effects of a number of influences, such as climate and lifestyle. These ideas are discussed in chapter three.

Exercise

This is sometimes known as gymnastics in Chinese texts. It is a system of gentle exercise in which Qi is guided by thought. Qi Gong and Tai Chi Chuan are the two main types, the latter being a variant of Qi Gong with the addition of various martial and longevity practices. They date back to at least the fourth century BC and are rooted in shamanism from a time when masters of wind and rain, fertility and death had a pre-eminent role in society. A number of simple Qi Gong exercises are described in chapter four.

Massage

This type of touch is one of the oldest methods of healing and can be practised by anyone, at virtually any time. Chinese massage allows Qi to flow smoothly in the body, strengthening it where it is weak, and dispersing it where it is blocked. It is similar to acupuncture in application and range of use, but uses finger pressure rather than needles to achieve the desired result. There are simple massage techniques described in chapter five.

Herbs

This, with acupuncture, is a stronger treatment and is traditionally used after other methods have failed. It involves the ingestion of powerful medicinal (herbal) substances which are individualized to suit the person and often mixed with other herbs to provide a balanced formula. However, if used incorrectly they have the potential to be harmful due to the strength of their effects, so they should always be treated with respect. With the correct formulation and administration they are beneficial to health and the removal of disease. The use of some simple herbal formulae and individual herbs (all of which are completely safe for self-administration) is described in chapter six.

Acupuncture

As with herbs, acupuncture is a stronger treatment, traditionally used when other methods have had little effect. It should always be carried out by a qualified practitioner; it is *not* a self-help treatment. It is a method of accessing Qi by the use of fine needles at specific points. Each point lies on a channel where the Qi flows through the body *(see page 24)*. The needle changes the flow of energy at that point, both in the channel and in its related organ. In this way, acupuncture can harmonize and strengthen Qi in the internal organs so that health is restored and symptoms are relieved. The professional application of acupuncture is described in chapter eight.

Astrology

Chinese astrology is a complex system of divination which can provide useful insights into your current situation and what life may hold in store for you. This allows you to judge the best course of action in a particular situation, offering insight into your personality and your psychological reactions. When we act according to what is most appropriate, our Qi flows harmoniously and we are healthy; Chinese astrology reveals the most appropriate course of action to take. *(See books listed on page 157 for more information.)*

Geomancy

This is known in Chinese as *feng shui* (literally 'wind and water'). It is a method of assessing the Qi of the environment which allows you to decide on the best place to site houses, working environments and so forth. It is taken very seriously by the Chinese: businesses, government organizations and individuals often determine the feng shui of buildings before working or living there.

When we live out of harmony with the Qi of the environment, it affects the Qi within our bodies, and symptoms and illness can result – for example 'sick building' syndrome: offices containing computers or machinery, with air-conditioning and little access to natural light, lead to employees being prone to colds, flu or even more serious diseases. *(For more information see recommended books on page 157.)*

SELF-HELP

The practicality of Chinese medicine is that it explains the functioning of the human body in simple language which is easy to understand. It is connected with simple observations which most of you have already made, although you may not realize it. For example, it explains why you feel a certain way when you eat a particular food or are in a particular climate. With a little knowledge, you can develop an understanding of how your body works, how it can be healthy and how you can minimize episodes of illness.

Limits to Self-help and Cautions

This book is not intended to replace the need to seek medical attention. The information given here is intended to help support health; it is not designed to offer medical diagnosis and treatment. If you have a symptom which is severe, getting progressively worse, limiting your activity or function or has come on rapidly over several hours, I would advise you to seek professional medical help. Chapter seven, which deals with specific symptoms, also contains clear information about when professional help is necessary.

ABOUT THIS BOOK

This book lays out the principles of Chinese medicine in a clear and practical way. It provides an ideal introduction to the world of Chinese medicine, whilst also offering self-help techniques that you can practise in your daily life, both for the relief of specific symptoms and to improve your health in general.

Beginning with a look at the origins and history of this ancient system of healing and how it spread to the West, the book goes on to discuss the underlying principles of Chinese medicine in chapter two. These principles are based on age-old observations, since found to be invaluable in understanding humans and their surrounding environments.

Chapters three to six offer self-help methods of treatment that will support your health and help you to deal with any symptoms that you may have. These chapters feature meditation, diet and lifestyle, Qi Gong exercises, massage techniques and herbal medicine. Chapter seven covers common symptoms and includes a fully comprehensive chart which enables you to discover, quickly and easily, the range of treatment options available for each specific symptom. The chart is fully cross-referenced with the information in chapters three to six so that you can turn to the details on the relevant method of treatment straight away. Advice on when to seek professional help is also given for each symptom.

The book concludes with information on practitioners of Chinese medicine: their training, how they practise, the methods of treatment they use and how to find a competent practitioner should you require one. Plus there is advice on what to look for if you are thinking of training in Chinese medicine yourself. Details of recognized societies, teachers and practitioners are given on page 157.

By reading this book you will be able to learn how to look at the world in a slightly different way to understand health and disease, and you will also learn practical skills which you can use to promote your own health and that of your family and friends.

CHAPTER ONE

ORIGINS AND HISTORY

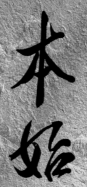

- *Evolution of Chinese medicine*
- *Classic texts and prominent figures in the field*
- *Chinese medicine today*
- *Spread across Asia and introduction to the West*
- *Continuing the tradition*

Chinese philosophical thought, of which Chinese medicine is merely one part, is a vast body of knowledge. It originates from a time when magic, spiritual practices, incantations and spells were very much an important part of people's lives. Today, many people see such things as superstition or without foundation, but in cultures which are much more connected with the earth and a sense of the supernatural their true value is still recognized.

ORIGINS OF CHINESE MEDICINE

Archaeological evidence has revealed the existence of acupuncture needles as far back as 1000 BC, and there have been discoveries of references to yin–yang theory in ancient texts of the same era. In fact, aspects of Chinese medicine can be found in a number of ancient texts, with the first recorded references to the five elements dating back to the Warring States Period of 476–221 BC.

The oldest textbook still in use in Chinese medicine is the 'Yellow Emperor's Inner Classic' (*Huangdi Neijing*) which was written about 300 BC and is still used as a source of information in schools of Chinese medicine. Parts of it are certainly much older, possibly by several thousands of years. The Yellow Emperor ruled over a loose collection of Chinese tribes about 2700 BC, and the book is written in the form of a dialogue between the Yellow Emperor and his chief minister, Qi Bo. It consists of two parts: 'Simple Questions' deals with general theories of medicine whilst 'Spiritual Axis' concentrates upon acupuncture. The *Neijing*, as it is known, is considered the 'bible' of Chinese medicine; it contains information from much

earlier texts and reveals the source of Chinese philosophy to be rooted in Taoist mysticism and shamanistic practices.

Many texts have since been written which are also still available to both students and practitioners. The 'Classic of Difficulties' (*Nanjing*) dates from around the first or second century AD. It contains information about the theory and practice of acupuncture. Written in a different style to the 'Yellow Emperor's Inner Classic', it reflects the change from a shamanistic tradition to the one which we now see today.

Two well-known figures in Chinese medicine date from around this period also. Hua Tuo was an eminent Taoist practitioner who developed various methods of treatment as well as Qi Gong exercises. Zhang Zhong Jing wrote the 'Discussion of Cold-induced Disorders' (*Shang Han Lun*) which is still in use today and is especially relevant to understanding diseases caused by climatic factors entering the body. He also developed several well-known herbal formulae, including Rehmannia Eight (*Jin Gui Shen Qi Wan – see page 120*) to treat disorders of the Kidney and

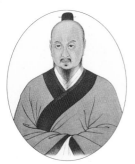

ZHANG ZHONG JING
(AD 150–219)

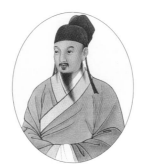

SUN SIMIAO
(AD 581–682)

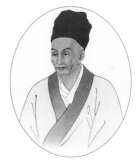

LI ZHI ZHEN
(AD 1518–1593)

wrote the classic herbal text, 'Prescriptions from the Golden Cabinet' *(Jingui Yaolue Fang)*.

Buddhist influences began to affect Chinese medicine around AD 600 and are particularly prominent in the works of Sun Simiao who lived at this time. He was known as the 'King of Medicine' because of his insights into Chinese herbal medicine and the treatment of women and children.

The Song dynasty 'Illustrated Manual on Points for Acupuncture and Moxibustion Shown on a Bronze Figure' *(Tongren Zhuxue Zhenjiu Tujing)*, written in the eleventh century AD, was followed by the special casting of two life-size bronze figures showing all the acupuncture points. The holes corresponding to the acupuncture points were sealed with wax, the models filled with water and correct needling of the points would result in the appearance of a flow of water. Quite an impressive teaching aid!

In the sixteenth century, the Ming dynasty physician, Li Zhi Zhen, wrote a herbal materia medica cataloguing the actions and uses of many herbs still used today. His pulse diagnosis classic is also very much used by students and practitioners of the present day: pulse diagnosis is an important method of diagnosis in Chinese medicine and has developed into a precise and refined art *(see page 151)*.

Later centuries, certainly in the last 150 years or so, have been marked in China by great social and political upheaval, and this has also affected the practice of medicine. In the earlier part of the twentieth century, Western conventional medicine began to be favoured as it was considered to be 'civilized and sophisticated', and until the Communist revolution of 1949, traditional Chinese medicine was in danger of suffering irreparable damage.

This unique Song-dynasty teaching aid enabled students to learn the correct needling of the acupuncture points. If a flow of water did not appear, the point had been needled incorrectly.

The fundamental aspects of Chinese medicine have been in practice for at least 4,000 years, and the particular type and style of treatment has changed in the light of experience and different cultural influences. Chinese medicine today is the result of this rich combination of theory and practice, ideas and experience. It continues to develop as new influences are brought to bear, most notably from its interaction with the West.

DEVELOPMENT IN CHINA

The history of Chinese medicine in China is long and illustrious. Over the centuries, there have been numerous influences and schools, each of which has placed a slightly different emphasis on particular aspects of treatment. For example, in the latter part of the twelfth century there was an emphasis on strengthening the digestive system, the 'gastrosplenic strengthening' school. In the sixteenth century there was the 'yang strengthening' school and during the seventeenth to eighteenth centuries, the 'hot diseases' school came into prominence. Clearly, this is partly to do with cultural changes in China itself, but it also reflects the changing patterns of disease; the disease of one generation is not the disease of the next. Patterns change as do lifestyle, living conditions and psychological states.

The different schools of influence have led to a rich and varied tradition of treatment which continues to the present day. Practitioners skilled in shamanistic and spiritual practices rooted in the origins of Chinese medicine practise alongside more 'conventional' practitioners. And then you have practitioners in the West whose different backgrounds influence the style of their practise. This shows that there is not one 'right' way of practising Chinese medicine, although the theoretical principles always remain the same.

CHINESE MEDICINE TODAY

In the People's Republic of China, there has been a particular emphasis on the practice of Chinese medicine since the Communist revolution of 1949. In the first half of the century, Western medicine was becoming the dominant form of medicine. Chinese medicine was in disarray and was seen as being primitive and unsophisticated; because of a lack of state support, it was in danger of falling into disuse. When the Communist government came into power, it was decided that Chinese medicine offered a practical, simple and affordable system of health care which could be applied to all sections of the population. Since then, it has been government policy to encourage and support traditional Chinese medicine and, as a consequence, Chinese medicine is now flourishing in China. This has spilled over into neighbouring countries, and Korea and Japan have also seen a revitalization of traditional medicine.

This has lessons for the West, where countries are weighed down by the funding of expensive, technological systems of medicine. Methods such as those available to Chinese medicine are not only cheap but also effective, and frequently remove the need for more expensive intervention.

However, there is a downside to the rejuvenation of Chinese medicine in China. The Communist government has presented it in a particular way to suit their ideological beliefs, with an emphasis on materialistic ideas while spiritual influences have been suppressed. This is still the case today, with cycles of relative freedom interspersed with savage control. Years of political and religious suppression in China have had the effect of making it very difficult for people to practise and study deeper ideas of the spirit. Consequently, many masters of Chinese medicine fled China after the revolution to settle in Taiwan, Korea and further afield. It is probably true to say that the deeper aspects of Chinese medicine are now more readily available in these countries and in the West than in their country of origin. A parallel situation has existed with Tibetan Buddhism, which was brutally suppressed by the Chinese after they invaded Tibet in 1959. It now flowers in India and in the West, and yet it is difficult to practise fully and freely in Tibet.

All of this has influenced the type of Chinese medicine which has reached the West. So-called Traditional Chinese medicine (TCM) is a result of the deliberate stripping of spiritual links from the body of Chinese medicine. This has not been completely successful and most practitioners and students have developed ways of overcoming this problem. They may seek training in other places such as Taiwan, Korea, Japan or Vietnam (although since 1975 the situation there has been somewhat similar to that of mainland China). The power of Chinese medicine is such that it works on a practical level to relieve common symptoms such as headaches, backache, diarrhoea and cough, for example, but it also addresses psychological disturbances and feelings of despair, disinterest and alienation which are now so pervasive in the West.

SPREAD ACROSS ASIA

Chinese medicine spread outwards from its origins within China as contacts developed with neighbouring countries. Buddhist monks were commonly responsible for transmitting such medicine to other oriental countries. This has heavily influenced Chinese medicine itself, and underlies the intimate connection between matters of the spirit and those of the physical body. With their vows of compassion and a commitment to help all sentient beings, the medicine practised by Buddhist monks reflected such concerns.

In each of the countries to which Chinese medicine spread, a native system of medicine was often already in existence, and this was consequently influenced and enriched by such contact. This has resulted in the practice of methods of medicine unique to the country concerned, and yet based upon the fundamental principles of Chinese medicine.

JAPAN

The traditional system of medicine already present in Japan was based upon purification by bathing, spiritual practices to drive out harmful spirits and on herbal medicine. Some elements of this remain, particularly bathing with the use of hot springs (a method used all over the world) and Shinto and Buddhist healing methods.

Japan was exposed to influences from Korean medicine from the fifth century AD onwards, but the spread of Chinese medicine directly from China began in the seventh century. Buddhist monks went to China and returned with Chinese medicine in addition to Buddhist studies. In AD 808, the first Japanese text on medicine was published: this 'Classified Collected Prescriptions of Great Unity' (*Daidō ruijûhō*). The 'Essential Medical Methods' (*Ishinpō*) by Tambo no Yasuyori, published in AD 984, is recognized as an essential continuation of the lineage of traditional Chinese medicine. It uses Buddhist ideas and Taoist practices.

KOREA

Due to the close proximity of Korea to China, its culture and system of medicine have been heavily influenced by its neighbour. Chinese medicine began to flow into Korea certainly by AD 100, during the Koguryô

China and the main Eastern countries (present day) to which the principles and methods of Chinese medicine spread. Those countries discussed in the text are highlighted in bold.

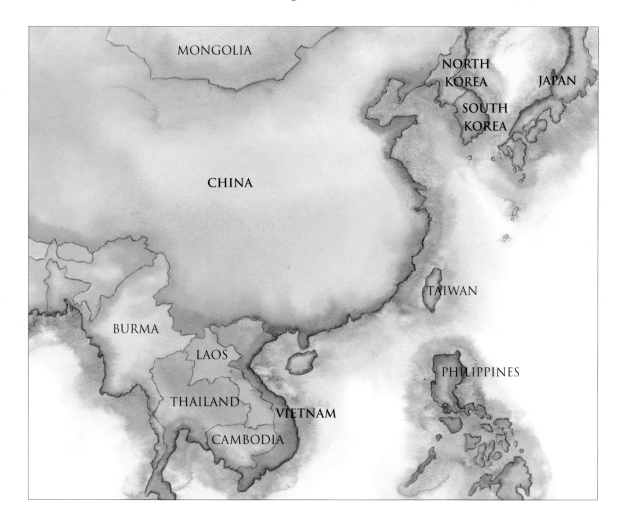

Dynasty. However, the Koreans themselves sought to modify such knowledge in the light of their own experience and the local environment. In addition, they combined it with indigenous medical practices. Korea was also influenced by Indian medicine during the fourth to seventh centuries AD because of connections through Buddhist monks.

Many texts were published in Korea over the centuries, none more influential than the twenty-five-volume 'Precious Mirror of Eastern Medicine' (Tongûi pogam) in 1631. This text is still studied in Korea. It drew upon previous texts such as the 'Yellow Emperor's Inner Classic', as well as local experience.

After Western medicine had been introduced to Korea, its traditional system of medicine came under threat. This, combined with foreign domination, particularly from Japan, served almost to eradicate such medicine by the 1940s. Since then, there has been a resurgence similar to that enjoyed by traditional medicine in China.

VIETNAM

There are two distinct strands of Vietnamese medicine. The oldest, 'Southern Medicine' (Thuoc nam), originated over 4,500 years ago and is indigenous to this area. It is based upon treatments by acupuncture, herbal formulae and diet. 'Northern Medicine' (Thuoc bac), on the other hand, is Chinese in nature and developed later, dating from 179 BC when Vietnam was ruled by China. Vietnam, conversely, influenced Chinese medicine in turn by the importation of Vietnamese herbs into China.

Over the intervening centuries, each strand of medicine (Northern and Southern) has continued its own course but also exerted influences over the other. What is now known as Traditional Vietnamese Medicine contains elements of both. The application of medicine was also tailored to meet the particular environment of Vietnam which is hot and damp with monsoons. There have also been close connections with spiritual practice, as in China, with Buddhism being the most obvious.

The eighteenth century Vietnamese physician, Hai Thuong Lan Ong Le hun Trac, wrote many texts but one in particular – his 'Treatise on Medical Knowledge' (Hai Thuong y tong tam linh) – is considered to be a great work and is still frequently used by students and practitioners today.

EAST MEETS WEST

There have been contacts between oriental culture and the West over many centuries. This can be seen in influences in Western art, pottery, science and now medical practice. Although Western conventional medicine has not been influenced by Chinese medicine, many Westerners have trained in China and other Eastern countries, and returned to the West to treat patients, bringing Eastern methods with them.

Some of the first contacts with Chinese culture were made by Jesuit priests and employees of the Dutch East India Company. A text on acupuncture and moxibustion (the burning of an aromatic dried herb, mugwort, to warm specific points and thereby increase energy, induce relaxation and relieve pain) was published in the West by the Dutch physician Willem ten Rhijne in 1683, and a number of other texts on Chinese medical theory were written by Jesuit missionaries in Japan about the same time.

Over the centuries, Chinese communities have lived in various different countries, practising Chinese medicine among themselves. However, the communities were rather insular so there was little contact with mainstream Western culture and thought. The main impact of Chinese medicine in the West was made after the 1960s (China was very much closed to Western contact and influences during the cultural revolution). In 1972, President Nixon and his staff, during a visit to China, observed the use of acupuncture anaesthesia. This clearly caused quite a stir, and subsequent contacts have brought Chinese medicine more into general Western consciousness.

Training courses have now been established in the People's Republic of China and many Western practitioners of Chinese medicine have trained either there or in other oriental countries. Also, many practitioners from China and neighbouring countries have moved to the West.

In recent years, numerous colleges have been set up in the West and it is now common to find practitioners in most towns. There are currently thousands of acupuncturists in the West, and other methods such as herbs, Qi Gong, massage and dietary therapy, although less commonly found, are increasing in popularity as each year passes. It is now possible for most people in the West to conveniently obtain treatment by means of Chinese medicine.

LINEAGE

Traditionally, the ideas and practices of Chinese medicine were handed down from generation to generation through a system of master to student. Each student would study and practise with a master of Chinese medicine and realize the truth of the teachings for themselves. After this period of learning, they would then become a master and, in turn, pass these teachings on to the next generation.

This idea of a lineage is an essential concept in oriental thought. Similarly, in Buddhism, teachings and spiritual practices can be traced back through a line of masters from the present day to the Buddha himself. The same is true in Taoism and, to some extent, in Chinese medicine, where teachings can be traced back to an original source. This tradition of master and student, which endures in an almost continual cycle, has

ensured that teaching and practice are interwoven, retain purity and yet remain fresh and dynamic.

Such methods of teaching Chinese medicine have become less common since the Communist revolution and the increasing tendency to use Western methods of training. The challenge for Western practitioners is to connect with these ancient teachings and their spiritual basis, and realize their truth for themselves.

In order to continue the benefits of Chinese medicine which have already been experienced for more than 4,000 years, we have a great responsibility to learn the theories and practices in their entirety and then to transmit these clearly, so that Chinese medicine not only takes root in the West, but can also go on to develop in succeeding generations.

QI
BODY ENERGY

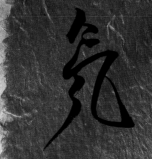

- The fundamental principles
  of Chinese medicine
  - Yin and yang
  - Qi as a 'life-force'
  - Causes of illness
- Channels and points of
  energy in the body
- The five elements and organs
  central to Chinese medicine

The essential point of Chinese medicine is that Qi, energy, flows throughout the body. It flows through channels and passes to the internal organs, and, together with Blood, it supplies nourishment to the body and ensures its normal functioning. We are healthy when Qi and Blood — the basis of life — are balanced within the body, and so flow harmoniously. Qi and Blood are aspects of yang and yin respectively, and to understand exactly how they affect our health we need to look first at how yin and yang fit into Chinese medicine as a whole.

YIN AND YANG

The words yin and yang are commonly heard today; they underlie all aspects of Chinese philosophy and medicine. They represent a different way of viewing the world compared to Western philosophy, yet allow great insights to be made about ourselves, the environment and our interactions with it. Yin and yang are the fundamental principles at the core of all existence; they represent the duality which is obvious in our everyday reality. The Chinese have used such ideas to develop a system of medicine which can effectively treat a wide range of disorders. This is why Chinese medicine is so effective: it is a *complete* system which has a *complete* view of the human being and of the universe, and as such it has many applications.

It is when one or other aspect of yin or yang is emphasized to the detriment of the other that imbalance becomes apparent. In the West there is often an emphasis on yang qualities of assertion, activity and achievement; when these are pursued without balance by yin qualities of receptivity and grounding, there is aggression, materialism and a tendency to flare up out of control. There is a Chinese saying that yang without yin is like a horse without reins, and yin without yang is cold and miserable. Yin and yang are inseparable and interdependent, and are therefore of equal value. This means that an extreme position of either yin or yang is inherently unbalanced: this can only lead to symptoms and ill-health.

The well-known symbol pictured above indicates the indivisibility yet interdependence of yin and yang. There is no situation where there is absolute yin or absolute yang: all parts of the universe are connected with each other as each object is in a state of constant change and interplay between these two opposite poles.

YIN AND YANG CHARACTERISTICS

Yin: *material, matter, structure, descent, below, cold, feminine, passive, contraction, interior, earth, water*

Yang: *immaterial, energy, function, ascent, above, hot, masculine, active, expansion, exterior, heaven, fire*

DUALITY AND ONENESS

Oneness, unity, is a spiritual level which transcends our mundane, everyday existence. It is the primordial state with which we are constantly striving to connect. Many spiritual paths exist to facilitate this; in China, the pre-eminent paths have been those of Taoism and Buddhism. Both date back to historical figures who lived around 500 BC, and the ideas they contain are even older. Meditation plays a large part; some simple exercises to practice are given in chapter three.

All the great religions and spiritual masters tell us that it is our duty to realize our innermost nature, our 'oneness'. In terms of Chinese philosophy, it is to transcend the duality of yang and yin, heaven and earth, yet at the same time our contact with the earth grounds us and reminds us of our mortality, humanity. In Chinese culture, there has always been a close link between spiritual and medical practice because of the recognition of the connectedness of all things, as seen in the ideas of yin and yang.

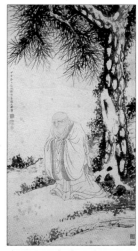

Lao-Tzu, the legendary founder of Taoism.

WHAT IS QI?

The active principle which results from the yin/yang dynamic is Qi. It is loosely translated as energy, although there is no direct counterpart in conventional Western thought. Qi takes particular forms in certain places at certain times; what we normally perceive as solid physical structures are nothing more than the concretization of energy. In Chinese teachings it is said, 'When Qi gathers, so the physical body is formed; when it disperses, so the body dies'. Qi is the life-force upon which the physical body depends. Therefore, in Chinese medicine, a person's health is dependent on three factors:

• The smooth flow of Qi and Blood.
• Good quality Qi and Blood.
• Correct functioning of the organs.

Since Qi is regarded as the life-force, it follows that the organs of the body must be understood from the perspective of Qi. In recognition of this role, by convention (in Chinese medicine texts in the West) the initial letter of organs and terms which refer to specific processes or entities in Chinese medicine are always capitalized (for example, Blood, Heat, and Yin and Yang when referring to a particular organ). This is to distinguish the complete energetic view of Chinese medicine from the physical organs of conventional Western medicine; an organ is likened to a particular sphere of action rather than just a physical structure. For example, the 'Kidney' in Chinese medicine is not merely the two physical organs situated in the lower part of the abdomen but is the general area of function, which includes the lower back, pelvis and reproductive system, and the knees and bones. It also supports the energy of all the other organs.

THE ROLE OF QI

Qi, with Blood, flows through channels which pass on the surface of the body as well as plunging deep within it to connect with internal organs and give life to the whole body. There are twelve main channels within the body, each associated with a particular organ, and there are 'points' along each channel which allow the practitioner to access the Qi and treat a disorder of that organ (*for more information on channels and points, see page 24*).

In addition to Qi, the Blood and bodily fluids also have an important role to play in maintaining health; the chart below outlines the main functions, disorders and associated symptoms for each.

QI, BLOOD AND FLUIDS: FUNCTIONS AND DISORDERS

Substance	Function	Disorder	Symptoms
Qi	Warms the body; provides the energy to drive metabolic functions; protects against invasion by climatic factors (and bacteria or viruses); holds fluids in their correct place. The Lung, Spleen and Kidney are the most important organs in ensuring strong, healthy Qi. The Liver ensures the smooth flow of Qi.	Weakness due to illness, poor diet, weak constitution, overwork and ageing	Weakness, tiredness, chilly feelings and specific symptoms of the organ affected
		Obstruction to smooth flow of Qi due to emotional upset, climatic influences, dietary factors and injury	Local pain and swelling. There may be symptoms of emotional disturbance
		'Rebellious' Qi (does not flow in a normal direction)	Stomach: nausea or vomiting; Lung: wheezing, cough; Spleen: prolapse
Blood	Cools the body; fluid, receptive and nourishing, particularly to the muscles and joints. Blood is a more material form of Qi. The Heart, Liver and Spleen are the most important organs in ensuring strong, healthy Blood.	Weakness due to heavy blood loss or reduced production of Blood, often associated with poor diet or weak digestive system	Dizziness, palpitations, pale skin, insomnia, anxiety, floaters in the vision, dry skin and hair
		Interrupted flow due to obstructed flow of Qi unable to circulate the Blood sufficiently, Cold or Heat affecting the Blood, or injury	Dark and dull complexion, purplish lips and tongue, painful swellings, fixed stabbing pain, and bleeding which is purple, black or clotted. There may be bruising
		Heat	Bright-red bleeding and rashes. In more severe cases there are mental symptoms of restlessness, delirium and coma
Fluids	Moisten, lubricate and provide nourishment to the body. Fluids include sweat, saliva and digestive juices; there are also fluids found in joints, the brain and spinal cord.	Loss due to high or long-lasting fever, profuse sweating, excessive urination, diarrhoea and vomiting	Dry mouth and thirst
		Accumulation	Swelling of legs, fingers or eyelids, cough with frothy, white sputum

HEALTH AND DISEASE

Chinese medicine has a positive view of health. When Qi and Blood are balanced and flow harmoniously through the body, the channels and the internal organs, it results in mental, emotional and physical well-being and vitality. Any departure from this state is, therefore, disease and there are many factors which may cause this.

It is important to note that a complete state of balance is somewhat idealized. There are clearly limitations placed upon us by our lifestyle, inherited characteristics and our reactions to our surroundings. Therefore, we should not consider balance to be a perfect state that we should struggle to attain by living 'perfect' lives, but rather consider life itself to be a process whereby we take ideas of Qi and Blood into account in adjusting our lifestyle and aspirations.

IMBALANCE IN QI AND BLOOD

According to Chinese texts, if Blood and Qi fall into disharmony 'a hundred diseases may arise'. Imbalances lead to symptoms and feelings of discomfort within the body and mind.

There are many possible combinations of imbalances affecting different organs. The art of Chinese medicine is to determine the exact nature of the imbalance and the best way to treat it for each *individual* person. Practitioners assess the balance of energy in three ways: by asking about the symptoms; by feeling the pulse; and by looking at the tongue. Further information is obtained by observing the face and complexion, or sometimes by physical examination. A diagnosis can then be made and treatment applied (*see chapter eight for further information on professional methods of diagnosis*).

Causes of imbalance

There are a number of factors which affect the balance of Qi and Blood, both inherited and environmental.

Constitution

Our inherited constitution (the strength of our Qi and Blood when we are born), is said to be dependent upon several factors:
- The health of our parents generally.
- Their health at the time of conception.
- Their age at the time of conception.

We tend to be stronger and healthier if our parents are generally well, were not suffering from any illness or disease at the time of conception and were relatively young; the early twenties is considered to be the best age to have children (though not always ideal). The baby's health may also be affected if conception occurs when the parents are intoxicated or excessively tired; the mother's health during pregnancy can be affected by drugs (prescribed or recreational) and by emotional shocks.

Climatic influences

The five main types of climatic factor which gain entry into the body are wind, cold, heat, damp and dryness; a sixth factor, summer-heat (extreme heat), may affect the body in summer. One or more factors (for example, WindHeat) may gain entry only when we are already weakened in some way or 'under the weather'. Where we live and the time of year largely determine the predominant climatic factors. For example, in Ireland cold and damp are found, and in Arizona heat and dryness. Each of the five main climatic factors is associated with a particular element, its corresponding organ and a season (*see pages 30–41*).

Imbalance in children

After birth, our environment plays a large part in our health. Babies are mainly affected by diet; the use of cow's-milk products, early weaning and the use of drugs and vaccinations may lead to ill-health. Diet is discussed in more detail in chapter three, and advice on a healthy diet for children is given on page 54.

Children are easily and commonly affected by emotional upsets, particularly within the family. In today's society, there is an increasing tendency to sexualize children early and present them with images which they can really only deal with when older. If children come into contact with such influences too young, it may lead to an imbalance in Qi and Blood.

Growing children have young and immature muscles and bones which are nourished by Blood. Excessive physical activity, especially in females at puberty, may lead to disturbances in the Blood which can manifest as menstrual difficulties, such as painful or irregular periods. Also, sexual activity at too early an age may disturb the balance of Qi and Blood. Maturity is considered to be around eighteen years of age. These observations about sexual activity and maturity are not moral judgements but the result of centuries of close study by Chinese medical practitioners who deeply understand the inner energies of the body. (See advice below left on bringing up a child.)

Imbalance in adults

With adults, diet, constitution and climatic influences are still important, but our emotions are even more involved in our health and how we feel. Anger, excessive joy, worry, overthinking or excessive study, sadness, fear and shock may all affect the flow of Qi in the body. Each emotion is related to a particular internal organ (see pages 31–41) and an excess of an emotion may adversely affect the organ or result from an organ imbalance. For example, grief is the emotion of the Lung: a bereavement or separation may lead to Lung symptoms – it is a common observation that the death of a partner may lead to pneumonia or bronchitis. Conversely, an imbalance in Lung energy may manifest as a sense of sadness.

Our daily lives, work and rest, are constant reminders of the factors which may affect us. Overwork and tiredness deplete the body's energy: short-term this may not be a problem as it can be replenished by rest, but long-term imbalances of internal organs may develop as they are put under strain to provide Qi and Blood in greater quantities. Our constitution governs our health in later life: if our inherited health is good, we are less likely to suffer from disease and associated symptoms later on; if it is poor, we may develop problems earlier.

RECOMMENDATIONS FOR BRINGING UP A HEALTHY CHILD

- *Do not expose your child to extremes of cold or heat.*
- *Do not carry your child all the time – lack of contact with the earth leads to shyness and fear.*
- *Do not overdress when playing.*
- *Keep back and stomach warm to protect Stomach and Kidney energy, and hands and feet warm to protect Heart and Lung energy.*
- *If there are hot feelings at the back of the neck, remove some clothes or your child may get a fever the next day.*
- *Massage your child regularly. The massage routine on pages 100–101 is beneficial for your child's health.*
- *Pay attention to diet: a healthy diet for children and babies is discussed on page 54.*
- *Do not overbathe.*
- *Do not expose your child to adult stress or arguments.*

LEVELS OF ENERGY

Qi flows both deep within the body and near the surface through 'channels', also known as *meridians*. There are places on each channel, 'points', where Qi can be accessed so that disturbances both in the channel and the internal organs can be treated. Symptoms of channel disturbances include pain, stiffness and swelling. Deep within the body, Qi flows within and between the organs. Disturbances here lead to symptoms inside the body, such as diarrhoea or cough; the symptoms depend upon the particular organ affected.

CHANNELS

The channels carry Qi, Blood and fluids around the body. The flow of Qi can be experienced during meditation practice, Qi Gong or when having treatment with acupuncture and massage. The sensation of Qi flowing along a particular channel or between different areas of the body is felt. There are twelve major channels in the body providing a constant flow of Qi and Blood to the organs (*see page 30 for the five main organs*) and to the exterior of the body. Each organ is paired with another organ, as are the channels (*see box below*). In this way, Lung points can be used

to treat the Large Intestine, and so forth. This principle also applies to herbal medicine (discussed in chapter six): for instance, herbs affecting the Stomach can be used to treat disorders of the Spleen. (Note: the points on the twelve main channels are featured with the relevant organs on pages 31–41.)

There are also eight other channels which allow for overflow when there is an abundance of Qi and Blood. These so-called 'Extra' channels have a role to play in Qi Gong and advanced meditation practices. Two are regularly used in clinical practice – the Conception Vessel (CV) and the Governor Vessel (GV) – and their points are listed on page 29.

Channels can provide information about the organ related to a particular symptom. For example, headaches at the side of the head are frequently related to the Gall Bladder channel as it supplies this area of the head (*see pages 26–28*). In this way, the channels and points can be used to treat symptoms that may appear to be completely unrelated to the organ concerned. There are several methods of treatment which directly affect the channels, including acupuncture, massage by An Mo or Tui Na and Qi Gong.

POINTS

These are particular locations of energy along the channels. They are sometimes likened to locations along a stream or river; the water begins by seeping up to the surface and then tumbling along a stream on a hillside. As the flow of water becomes larger, it tends to slow down and form pools or lakes, and eventually the water reaches the sea. Similarly, the flow of energy at a particular point may be slow and calm, yet at others it may be forceful and

---

THE TWELVE MAIN CHANNELS
IN PAIRS

- *Lung* (Lu) *and Large Intestine* (LI)
- *Spleen* (Sp) *and Stomach* (St)
- *Heart* (H) *and Small Intestine* (SI)
- *Pericardium* (P) *and Triple Burner or* San Jiao (SJ)
- *Kidney* (K) *and Urinary Bladder* (UB)
- *Liver* (Liv) *and Gall Bladder* (GB)

rapid. Each point, therefore, has a different function, and treating different points has specific yet different effects.

The Chinese word for a point, *xue wei*, literally means 'hole/cave place', and this is what it feels like when you touch it. There may be an obvious physical depression or a sensation that the surface of the skin is somewhat different at that place. In China, the traditional way of referring to points is by their poetic names; each point has a personality of its own and this is encapsulated in its name – for example, 'Yang Pool', which is at the back of the neck where Wind (which is yang) collects before entering the body, or 'Hundred Meetings', which is at the top of the head where many channels meet. Western practitioners of Chinese Medicine tend to refer to the points as numbers on the channels: for example, GB20. There are, however, some points that can only be identified by name, since they are not allocated to a specific channel (where applicable, the number version is used when referring to points in the text).

Points can be used to access energy deep within the body. For example, the point St36 on the leg is related to the function of the Stomach, and massage or needling of this point will increase Stomach energy and harmonize the digestion. In China, this point is often massaged daily because strong Stomach energy is associated with long-life and health.

Specific points

There are a number of points mentioned in this book and they are referred to later on with regard to Qi Gong, massage and the self-help chapter on symptoms. At this stage it is helpful to begin to locate some points on yourself or your family and friends so that you can begin to learn where they are and

what they feel like. Although pages 26–28 clearly show where each point is located, do feel the area for yourself in order to appreciate any sensations you may experience while doing so. Points are frequently situated close to bony areas, skin creases and other identifiable marks. However, they can also be detected by feeling the energy on the surface of the body: an area may feel warm or cold; you may notice that a particular area feels 'different' to the surrounding area; or there may be some tenderness if the energy of the point is out of balance. As your experience grows, you should soon be able to find the locations of points on your own.

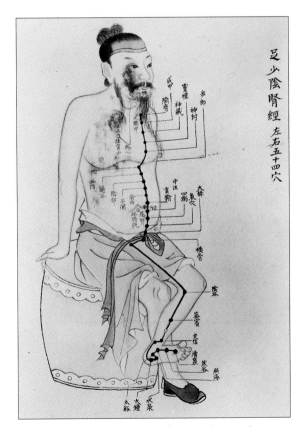

A traditional illustration of a seated man showing the Kidney channel and its points.

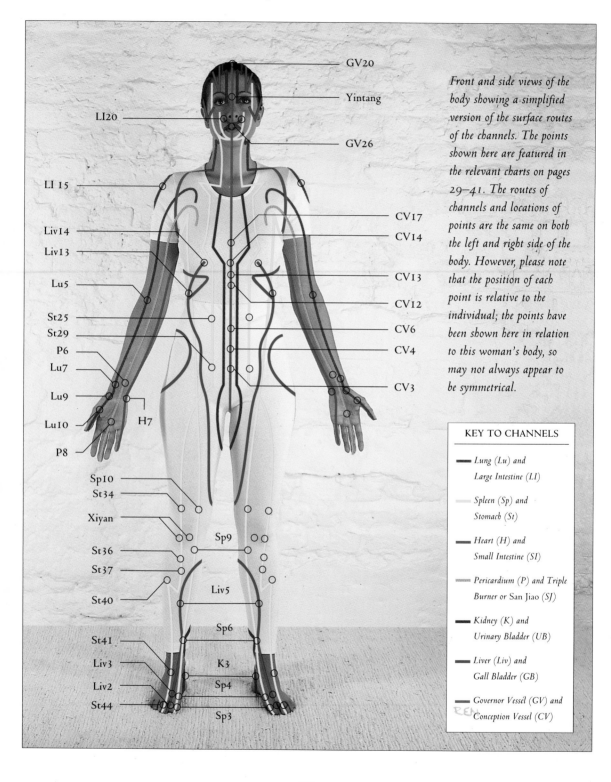

GV20

Yintang

LI20

GV26

LI 15

Liv14

Liv13

Lu5

St25

St29

P6

Lu7

Lu9

Lu10

P8

H7

CV17

CV14

CV13

CV12

CV6

CV4

CV3

Sp10

St34

Xiyan

Sp9

St36

St37

St40

Liv5

Sp6

St41

Liv3

K3

Liv2

Sp4

St44

Sp3

Front and side views of the body showing a simplified version of the surface routes of the channels. The points shown here are featured in the relevant charts on pages 29–41. The routes of channels and locations of points are the same on both the left and right side of the body. However, please note that the position of each point is relative to the individual; the points have been shown here in relation to this woman's body, so may not always appear to be symmetrical.

KEY TO CHANNELS

━━ *Lung (Lu) and Large Intestine (LI)*

━━ *Spleen (Sp) and Stomach (St)*

━━ *Heart (H) and Small Intestine (SI)*

━━ *Pericardium (P) and Triple Burner or San Jiao (SJ)*

━━ *Kidney (K) and Urinary Bladder (UB)*

━━ *Liver (Liv) and Gall Bladder (GB)*

━━ *Governor Vessel (GV) and Conception Vessel (CV)*

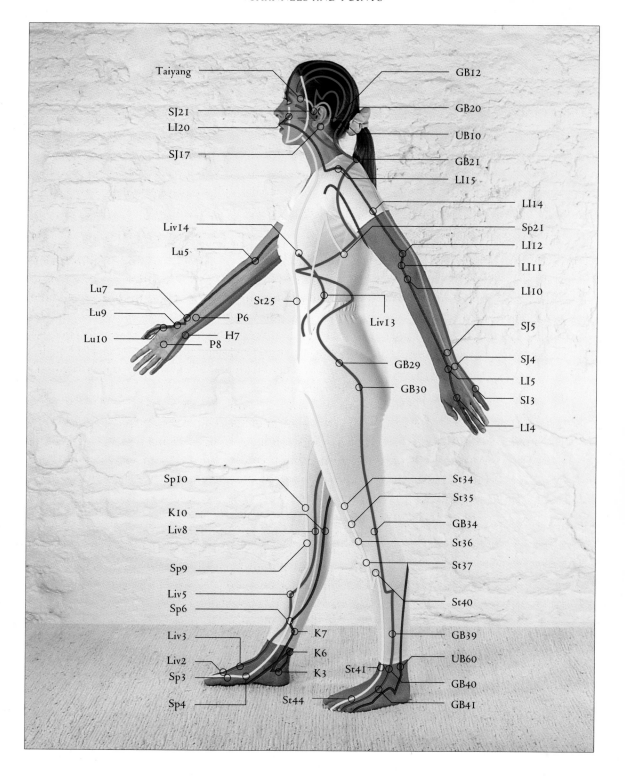

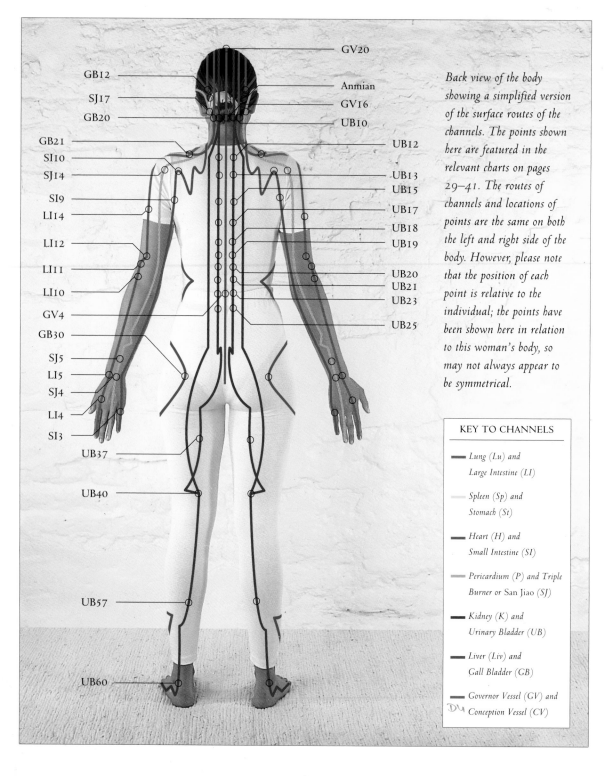

GV20

GB12
Anmian

SJ17
GV16

GB20
UB10

GB21
UB12

SI10

SJ14
UB13

SI9
UB15

LI14
UB17

UB18

LI12
UB19

LI11

LI10
UB20

UB21

GV4
UB23

GB30
UB25

SJ5

LI5

SJ4

LI4

SI3

UB37

UB40

UB57

UB60

Back view of the body showing a simplified version of the surface routes of the channels. The points shown here are featured in the relevant charts on pages 29–41. The routes of channels and locations of points are the same on both the left and right side of the body. However, please note that the position of each point is relative to the individual; the points have been shown here in relation to this woman's body, so may not always appear to be symmetrical.

KEY TO CHANNELS

Lung (Lu) and
Large Intestine (LI)

Spleen (Sp) and
Stomach (St)

Heart (H) and
Small Intestine (SI)

Pericardium (P) and Triple
Burner or San Jiao (SJ)

Kidney (K) and
Urinary Bladder (UB)

Liver (Liv) and
Gall Bladder (GB)

Governor Vessel (GV) and
Conception Vessel (CV)

POINTS ON THE 'EXTRA' CHANNELS

Points	Functions	Used to treat
FRONT OF TRUNK AND CHEST		
CV3 Central Pole*	Strengthens Kidneys, clears Heat and Dampness from the lower abdomen	Cystitis, vaginal discharge
CV4 Hinge at the Source*	Strengthens Kidneys	Low backache, impotence, urinary frequency
CV6 Sea of Qi*	Strengthens Kidneys, strengthens Qi	Vaginal discharge, diarrhoea
CV12 Central Stomach	Strengthens and regulates Spleen and Stomach, transforms Dampness and Phlegm	Indigestion, nausea, vomiting, tiredness, diarrhoea
CV13 Upper Stomach	Strengthens Stomach	Indigestion, nausea, bloated upper abdomen
CV14 Great Palace	Calms the Spirit, calms the Stomach	Anxiety, cough, vomiting
CV17 Central Altar	Regulates Lungs, strengthens Qi, relaxes the chest	Cough, tiredness, hiccups, anxiety
BACK		
GV4 Gate of Life	Strengthens Kidneys, regulates Water, warms the Yang, strengthens lower back and knees, strengthens *Jing* (Essence)	Disorders of periods, low back pain, frequent urination, incontinence, impotence
GV16 Wind's Palace	Disperses Wind, WindCold and WindHeat	Common cold, headache, heaviness in head, blocked nose
HEAD AND FACE		
Anmian (*not on specific channel*)	Calms the mind	Insomnia
Yintang: Original Cavity of the Spirit (*not on specific channel*)	Calms the Spirit, disperses WindHeat	Headache, anxiety, insomnia
Taiyang (Sun) (*not on specific channel*)	Disperses Wind, benefits the eyes	Headache at the side of the head, common cold
GV20 Hundred Meetings	Calms the Spirit, spreads Liver Qi	Faintness, tiredness and collapse, headache
GV26 Middle of Man	Clears senses, calms Spirit, helps lower back	Low back pain, shock

* Do not use during pregnancy

FIVE ELEMENTS · FIVE ORGANS

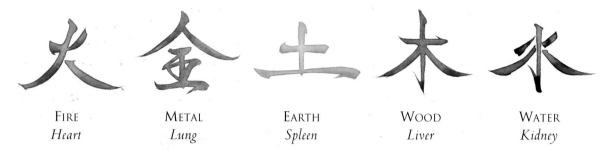

FIRE	METAL	EARTH	WOOD	WATER
Heart	*Lung*	*Spleen*	*Liver*	*Kidney*

The duality of yin and yang described earlier in this chapter is clearly not enough, by itself, to explain the totality of human experience. There are shades of yin and yang, of cold and heat, and such subtleties of meaning allow us to interpret our relationship with nature – the functioning of our body and mind and how we change with the seasons and time. Yet at the same time, yin and yang are the relative expression of our absolute nature – our oneness (*see below*).

The duality of yin and yang can be expanded to four elements which correspond to the four seasons. Each season represents a particular energy and, in Chinese medicine, the seasons are ascribed to the elements as follows: Wood (spring), Fire (summer), Metal (autumn) and Water (winter). This idea is common to many traditional systems of medicine and was prevalent in European philosophy during the Middle Ages. In Chinese medicine, there is the addition of a central phase (Earth) to form five elements.

At different times of the year, yin or yang becomes more prominent, and this is reflected in the seasons (*see below*). The most yang time is known as 'yang within yang' and corresponds to the height of summer. The most

UNITY

SPIRIT · GOD · BUDDHANATURE
*This gives rise to the duality of yin and yang,
the reality of everyday experience*

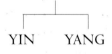

YIN   YANG

*The functioning energies of yin and yang reflect our
relationship with nature – how we are affected by the time
of day and time of year*

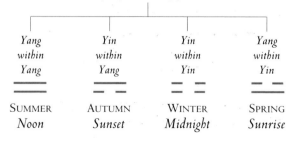

Yang within Yang	Yin within Yang	Yin within Yin	Yang within Yin
SUMMER	AUTUMN	WINTER	SPRING
Noon	*Sunset*	*Midnight*	*Sunrise*

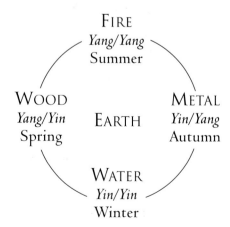

FIRE
Yang/Yang
Summer

WOOD
Yang/Yin
Spring

EARTH

METAL
Yin/Yang
Autumn

WATER
Yin/Yin
Winter

yin time is 'yin within yin' and corresponds to the height of winter. As the yin of winter subsides, the yang begins to burst forth into spring: this is the 'yang within yin'. Conversely, as the yang of summer wanes and draws within, autumn appears: this is 'yin within yang'.

Just as yin and yang can be expanded to the four elements, these, in turn, can be expanded to the *Ba Gua*. The Ba Gua has many meanings, and its use in Qi Gong is described in chapter four (*see pages 68–69*). Each expansion allows for further refining of the application of yin and yang (the original basis). The next stage is an expansion to the sixty-four hexagrams of the *I Ching*, or *Book of Changes*, used in the art of divination and relevant to the tradition of astrology mentioned at the beginning of the book on page 8.

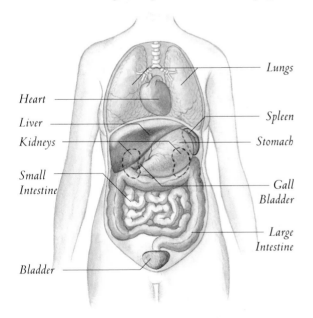

This illustration shows the positioning of the organs which correspond, in pairs, to the major channels of the body (see also page 24). The kidneys, represented here by a dotted line, are situated at the back of the rib-cage, behind the other organs.

This demonstrates the depth of Chinese medicine and the interconnections between its different aspects.

Each of the five elements is associated with an organ and area of the body, as well as with aspects of the natural world. In this way, it is possible to gain an understanding of the person's energy and its relationship with the natural environment. The five main organs that control activity and function within the body are the Heart, Lungs, Spleen, Liver and Kidneys, illustrated below left, along with their paired organs.

The rest of this chapter looks at the five main organs and elements in detail. For each organ, useful points located on the relevant channel pairing are given: refer to the illustrations on pages 26–28 for their location on the body.

You will find it helpful to return to the information in this section now and again, especially when referring to the symptoms in chapter seven. In this way, you will gradually incorporate the ideas of Chinese medicine into your everyday life.

FIRE • HEART

Fire conjures up ideas of heat, redness, brightness and activity. Consequently, it corresponds to the summertime and to midday, and is yang within yang. It is luxuriant and flourishing. The Heart is the organ which is associated with the Fire element.

The Heart actively pumps Blood around the body. It transforms Qi from food into Blood; it is said that 'The Heart stamps the Blood red'. The Heart houses consciousness and the mind; all our mental functions of thinking, memory and concentration, as well as sleep and dreams, depend upon a healthy Heart so that the mind is calm and relaxed.

Traditionally, two extra organs are associated with the Fire element to complete the twelve channels listed on page 24. Firstly, there is the Pericardium. This covers the Heart and protects it from outside influences such as emotional stresses and strains. It is closely connected with psychological states, and points on this channel are used to treat psychological disturbances. Secondly, the organ that is paired with the Pericardium is the Triple Burner (*San Jiao*). This is a connecting pathway through the body that deals with the movement of water. There is no related organ in Western medicine.

Disturbances of the Heart

Within the Heart, there is a yang (Qi) aspect and a yin (Blood) aspect. Heart Qi is to do with activity, and weakness of Heart Qi leads to tiredness, pallor, palpitations, cold extremities, sweating in the day, shortness of breath and discomfort in the chest. In more severe cases there will be water swelling in the legs and more cold feelings. Heart Blood anchors the Qi, and if weakened leads to an overactive mind. Symptoms associated with weak Heart Blood include anxiety, palpitations, insomnia, dream disturbed sleep, poor memory, pallor and dizziness. In severe cases where yin is affected, signs of heat appear such as night sweats, dry mouth and throat, and perhaps slight redness in the cheeks.

METAL · LUNG

Metal takes many forms, and in its natural state it is something that does not 'hold on' to things; things do not stick to metal, and so there is a natural function of letting go, of some form of separation. In Chinese medicine this element is associated with autumn: it is yin within the yang. The Lung is the

---

HEART ASSOCIATIONS

- **Colour:** *red. This is the colour of the Heart, of Blood. In the West, pharmaceutical companies mainly use red for tablets affecting the heart.*

- **Emotions:** *joy, love. Chinese brides frequently get married in red. Loneliness and separation affect the Heart energy, hence the terms 'broken heart', 'heartache'.*

- **Mental associations:** *The Heart is the 'Residence of the Mind' (Spirit or Shen). Attitudes such as gratitude, humility, appreciation and politeness originate here, hence a 'kind heart'. Points on the Heart channel may be used to treat disorders of the mind, such as confusion and delirium.*

- **Sense organ:** *tongue. Joy and love have to be communicated to become fully realized.*

- **Paired organ:** *Small Intestine. Emotional upset, particularly anxiety, may lead to diarrhoea.*

- **Taste:** *bitter. Excess bitter taste may affect Heart energy. Bitter-tasting herbs are usually used to treat excess Heat in the body.*

- **Time:** *11am–1pm. This is when Heart energy is strongest. Heart attacks are more common around noon if this strong energy becomes obstructed.*

- **Season:** *summer. This is the hottest, most yang time of the year and the time when nature is at its most active.*

- **Climate:** *heat. The Heart can be affected by fevers with symptoms such as delirium and palpitations. Heat may affect other organs, of course.*

---

main organ associated with the Metal element.

The Lung takes in Qi from the external environment. Inspiration, breathing in, may be considered from a spiritual context as an energizing, uplifting state which affects us

HEART, SMALL INTESTINE, PERICARDIUM AND TRIPLE BURNER CHANNELS

Points	Functions	Used to treat
H7 Spirit Gate	Strengthens and regulates Heart	Anxiety, insomnia
SI3 Back Stream	Relaxes sinews, helps joints, relieves pain	Low backache
SI9 True Shoulder	Helps the shoulder, disperses Wind	Pain in shoulder
SI10 Upper Arm Point	Helps the shoulder, disperses Wind	Pain in shoulder
P6 Inner Pass	Strengthens and regulates Heart, calms the Spirit, expands and relaxes chest and upper abdomen	Anxiety, insomnia, indigestion, nausea, vomiting, morning sickness, hiccups
P8 Palace of Labour	Regulates Heart	Fever, unconsciousness. Mainly used in Qi Gong practices and healing to absorb Qi from the universe and to direct it outwards
SJ4 Yang Pool	Disperses Wind	Sore throat, common cold, pain in wrist and forearm
SJ5 Outer Pass	Clears Heat, strengthens protective Qi, disperses Wind	Fever, pain in joints which moves around, common cold, deafness and tinnitus (ringing in ears), pain in wrist and forearm
SJ14 Shoulder Opening	Helps the shoulder	Pain and stiffness in shoulder
SJ17 Shielding Wind	Helps ears, disperses Wind and Cold	Deafness, tinnitus, earache, sore throat, toothache
SJ21 Ear Gate	Helps ears	Deafness, tinnitus, earache

deeply. On a physical level, it can simply be considered as the physical act of taking in air; in these modern times, when despair, depression and general lack of inspiration are common, it is clearly no coincidence that asthma is much more widespread. Air that is recycled, conditioned (or rather 'deconditioned'), polluted or stale provides us with less Qi to absorb. People who live in cities often suffer from Lung problems as a result.

The Lung also controls the surface of the body. This protects against the invasion of influences such as climatic factors, bacteria and viruses or emotional influences in the surrounding environment. Lung energy passes downwards and outwards and regulates the flow of Water in the body, especially the upper part; disruption of Water metabolism may result in no sweating, water retention, scanty urination or difficulty passing urine. The skin, sweat glands and body hair are also governed by the Lungs; Lung imbalances can lead to dry skin, increased sweating and greater vulnerability to external causes of disease.

Disturbances of the Lung

Within the Lung, there is a yang (Qi) aspect and a yin aspect, and symptoms differ according to which aspect is primarily affected. For example, Lung Qi resists the invasion of climatic factors. If a climatic factor does gain entry, the Lung responds by closing the pores to prevent further invasion, and there is then a struggle at the surface of the body between the person's Qi and that of the climatic factor. When this happens, typical symptoms are those of the common cold.

In other situations, weakness of Lung Qi leads to cough, breathlessness, pallor, tiredness and a weak voice. If it is complicated by the accumulation of Dampness (mucus) there will be sputum which may be white or yellow (see 'Dampness and Phlegm' on page 36). Weakness of Lung Yin (Water) leads to dry cough, night sweats, slight redness in the face, dry mouth and throat, thin body (weight loss if it is of recent development) and hot sensations in the palms of the hands and the soles of the feet. Any sputum is dry, scanty and hard to cough up due to the dryness.

EARTH · SPLEEN

Mother Earth nourishes and supports us. From birth, our mothers protect and nurture us, provide us with comfort and are central to our growth and development. Similarly, the associated organ of the Earth element, the Spleen, takes food into our bodies and transforms it into Qi to nourish and support all the other organs. If transformation does not occur, there is a churning over with rumbling in the abdomen, or thoughts which turn over in the mind and do not go anywhere.

The Spleen is the organ concerned with digestive function. Together with the Lungs, it provides the body with regular daily supplies

---

LUNG ASSOCIATIONS

• **Colour**: *white. In China, this is traditionally associated with death. Black, frequently used in the West, is a later development and almost certainly reflects our difficulty in dealing with death, since black is the colour of the Water element (see page 40) and is associated with fear.*

• **Emotion**: *grief, sadness. The Metal element has the characteristic of letting go, of things not holding on; things slide off metal objects. The Lungs and their paired organ, the Large Intestine, very much have a role in letting go.*

• **Mental associations**: *sensitivity, compassion, vulnerability and openness. An imbalance may result in over-sensitivity to external influences or the emotions of others. Conversely, there may be a lack of sensitivity.*

• **Sense organ**: *nose. Problems here may manifest as blocked nose, runny nose or reduced sense of smell.*

• **Paired organ**: *Large Intestine. In those of you who smoke or have done, this connection explains how smoking a cigarette can stimulate the bowels.*

• **Taste**: *spicy. Excess intake of spicy foods such as chillies and black pepper will damage the Lung.*

• **Time**: *3–5am. This is the time when the Lung energy is at its fullest. A cough with phlegm is frequently worst at this time.*

• **Season**: *autumn. This is when the energy starts to withdraw into the interior in readiness for the cold of winter.*

• **Climate**: *dry. The Lungs are moist and are easily affected by dryness.*

---

of Qi and, ultimately, Blood. Weakness in either organ, or poor quality food and air, will lead to weakening of the body in general. The role of food in our state of health and how it specifically affects different organs is

LUNG AND LARGE INTESTINE CHANNELS		
Points	Functions	Used to treat
Lu5 Cubit Marsh	Strengthens and regulates Lungs, clears Heat	Cough with sputum, sore throat, pain in elbow
Lu7 Broken Sequence	Regulates Lungs, disperses WindCold and WindHeat	Headache, common cold, cough, sore throat, pain in wrist, pain and stiffness in neck
Lu9 Great Abyss	Strengthens and regulates Lungs, clears Heat	Cough, sore throat
Lu10 Fish Border	Cools Heat in Lungs, benefits throat	Sore throat, hoarse voice
LI4 Union Valleys*	Disperses Wind, WindCold and WindHeat	Common cold, cough, headache, toothache, rash, blocked nose, runny nose
LI5 Yang Ravine	Dispels WindHeat, transforms DampHeat	Headache, toothache, pain in wrist
LI10 Arm Three Miles	Regulates Stomach and Intestines	Indigestion, diarrhoea, vomiting, pain in elbow
LI11 Curved Pool	Disperses Wind and WindHeat, clears Heat	Rash, pain in elbow, fever
LI12 Elbow Bone-hole	Benefits the elbow	Pain in the elbow and arm
LI14 Upper Arm's Musculature	Relaxes sinews	Pain in upper arm and shoulder
LI15 Shoulder Bone	Relaxes sinews, relieves shoulder	Pain and stiffness in shoulder
LI20 Welcome Fragrance	Opens the nose, disperses WindHeat	Blocked nose, runny nose, common cold

* Do not use during pregnancy

discussed in chapter three (see page 52).

Spleen Qi keeps Blood in the vessels; bruising or bleeding may result from weakness of Spleen Qi. It also holds organs in their place, and controls muscles and flesh. When Spleen Qi is strong the muscles are healthy, of good tone and strong; wasting of muscles may be a result of a Spleen Qi weakness.

Disturbances of the Spleen

Weakness of Spleen Qi tends to manifest as digestive disorders with symptoms of poor appetite, general tiredness and tiredness in the limbs, loose stools, sallow complexion and abdominal distension. In more severe cases there will be coldness and diarrhoea at four or five o'clock in the morning, so-called 'cock-crow' diarrhoea. In some people, the weakness of Spleen Qi mainly affects its function of raising organs, resulting in prolapse of the rectum or uterus. There may also be problems due to accumulation of Dampness (mucus) within the body, and these are discussed overleaf.

Dampness and Phlegm

A weakness in Spleen Qi results in less Qi being produced, but it also produces fluids which are thicker than normal. This is manifest as increased amounts of mucus in the body: in Chinese medicine, the technical term for this is Dampness. This either passes up into the Lungs, leading to cough with sputum, nasal discharge and heaviness in the head, or sinks down into the lower parts of the body, such as the Intestines, leading to mucus in the stools, vaginal discharge or urinary symptoms.

There is some relationship between Dampness inside the body and damp in the environment. When the climate is damp, Dampness is more likely to accumulate. When this Dampness is thicker it is known as Phlegm. This may be obvious as sputum coughed up from the Lungs, but may also manifest as swollen glands, a generally 'muzzy' feeling in the head or may even, in severe situations, lead to confusion, paralysis or tumours.

WOOD · LIVER

The Wood element is characterized by a tree in springtime, bursting forth with new growth and activity after the quiet of winter. The energy of spring ascends as new growth begins; the counterpart in human life is in childhood and around the time of puberty. The Liver is the organ associated with the Wood element. Green is the colour of new growth in nature and is the colour associated with the Liver. This is why children do not like green vegetables as they have a lot of this energy already!

The Liver ensures the smooth and harmonious flow of energy throughout the body and all of its organs. Pain and emotional

---

SPLEEN ASSOCIATIONS

• **Colour:** *yellow. This is the colour of Earth. Yellow foods which grow in the Earth are good at strengthening the Spleen and Stomach: these include parsnips, potatoes, carrots, squash and pumpkin (all generally sweet).*

• **Emotion:** *sympathy. If the Spleen is imbalanced there may be a lack of sympathy or an inability not to be sympathetic; being oversympathetic can deplete Spleen Qi.*

• **Mental associations:** *belief, faith, confidence and trust. The Spleen is the 'Residence of Thought': if Spleen Qi is weak, we may have difficulty with concentration and memory; if we overthink, we may deplete Spleen Qi. The Stomach relates to endurance and stamina; Stomach imbalance may lead to lack of patience or endurance.*

• **Sense organ:** *mouth. Mouth ulcers, sore gums, bleeding gums and toothache are often a result of a Stomach or Spleen imbalance.*

• **Paired organ:** *Stomach. The Stomach receives food and the Qi of the Spleen 'cooks' it. The Stomach is like a cooking pot with the Fire of the Spleen beneath it. This action of the Spleen results in food being transformed into Qi and fluids which are then transported to other parts of the body.*

• **Taste:** *sweet. Excess sweet taste will damage the Stomach and Spleen. A desire for sweet food indicates weak Spleen Qi.*

• **Time:** *7–11am for both Spleen and Stomach. Breakfast needs to be the largest meal of the day at the time when the Spleen and Stomach energy is full and flourishing. Try not to eat late at night when these organs need to rest.*

• **Season:** *the season of Earth is often described as late summer, but it is more useful to think of it as the centre, which reflects the central role of the Spleen and Stomach.*

• **Climate:** *damp. The Spleen is affected by damp climate. Spleen disturbances lead to the accumulation of Dampness within the body (see above left).*

SPLEEN AND STOMACH CHANNELS

Points	Functions	Used to treat
Sp3 Great White	Strengthens and regulates Spleen and Stomach, transforms Dampness and DampHeat	Poor appetite, nausea, vomiting, indigestion, diarrhoea, belching, constipation
Sp4 Yellow Emperor	Strengthens and regulates Spleen and Stomach, transforms Dampness and DampHeat	Indigestion, vomiting, diarrhoea
Sp6 Three Yin Junction*	Strengthens and regulates Spleen, transforms Dampness, spreads Liver Qi, strengthens Kidneys	Diarrhoea, cystitis, vaginal discharge, painful periods
Sp9 Yin Mound Spring	Strengthens and regulates Spleen, resolves Damp especially in lower abdomen and pelvis	Cystitis, vaginal discharge, knee pain
Sp10 Sea of Blood	Strengthens Blood, cools Heat	Anaemia, rash, itching
Sp21 Great Envelope	Relaxes chest, regulates flow of Qi and Blood through whole body	Generalized body aches and pains
St25 Heaven's Axis	Regulates Spleen and Stomach, transforms Dampness, regulates and moistens Intestines	Indigestion, constipation, diarrhoea
St29 Return*	Regulates menstruation, transforms DampHeat	Lower abdominal pain, painful periods, vaginal discharge
St34 Connecting Mound	Regulates Stomach, clears Heat	Pain and stiffness in knee
Xiyan *This is a pair of points on either side of the knee (one is St35 and the other is not on a specific channel).*	Helps the knee, disperses Wind and Cold, clears Heat	Knee pain
St36 Foot Three Miles	Strengthens and regulates Spleen and Stomach, transforms Dampness and DampHeat	Poor appetite, indigestion, tiredness, diarrhoea, cough with sputum, anaemia, pain and stiffness in knee
St37 Upper Great Hollow	Regulates Stomach and Intestines	Diarrhoea, constipation
St40 Bountiful Bulge	Regulates Stomach and Intestines, transforms Dampness and Phlegm, calms the Spirit	Cough with sputum, dizziness
St41 Separate Stream	Regulates Stomach	Headache, vomiting, indigestion
St44 Inner Courtyard	Regulates Stomach, transforms DampHeat, clears Heat	Hiccups, indigestion, toothache, sore throat

* Do not use during pregnancy

disturbances are common symptoms that arise if the Liver cannot smooth the flow of Qi through the body. The Liver also has a role to play in Blood metabolism: when we rest, particularly when lying down, Blood returns to the Liver and is stored there. This Blood is released during exercise and menstruation. In addition, the Liver is related to tendons; it is concerned with movement of the four limbs and governs smooth movement of the joints. The condition of our nails is connected to the Liver, as they are a 'by-product' of the sinews.

Disturbances of the Liver

The Liver is usually affected by obstruction to the free flow of Qi. Common causes of this are emotional upsets, which explains why Liver Qi obstruction is frequently seen in the modern world. Other factors are eating too much sweet and greasy food, injury and climatic factors (see page 22). Symptoms are seen where the Liver channel passes through the body, such as the breasts in women, the abdomen, genital area and eyes. The sides of the head may also be affected as this area is supplied by the Gall Bladder channel, which is paired with the Liver. There may be pre-menstrual symptoms of breast soreness, headache and irritability. Migraine-like headaches are associated with obstruction to the flow of Liver Qi also. Weakness of the Liver Blood causes floaters in the vision, numbness and tingling and may lead to a stirring of Liver Qi (Wind); this can manifest as tics and tremors.

WATER · KIDNEY

The Water element is fluid yet hides, within its depths, secrets and mysteries. The deep unconscious is associated with Water in many

---

LIVER ASSOCIATIONS

- **Colour:** *green. This is the colour of spring, of bile (which is produced in the Liver), and of envy and jealousy.*

- **Emotion:** *anger, irritability. Such emotions are a consequence of disturbance in the flow of Qi. Related emotions include resentment, fury, rage and jealousy. A healthy flow of Liver Qi is seen as assertiveness rather than aggression.*

- **Mental associations:** *a giving attitude and sharing. Overactivity of the Liver is associated with aggression and blaming others, whereas underactivity of the Liver is associated with lack of assertiveness and blaming oneself.*

- **Sense organ:** *eye. Liver disturbances may affect the eye, with symptoms such as migraine headaches and spots in the vision.*

- **Paired organ:** *Gall Bladder. Traditionally, the Liver was considered to be the 'General', in charge of planning and providing the overall control of activity. The Gall Bladder puts these plans 'into action', and so courage and decision-making are the realm of this organ.*

- **Taste:** *sour. Excess sour taste will damage the Liver. Sweet and sour foods are often found in Chinese cooking: the sweet taste strengthens the Spleen whilst the sour taste encourages the Liver to allow the free flow of Qi. In this way, digestion is aided and function is not obstructed.*

- **Time:** *1–3am. Difficulty getting to sleep is a consequence of obstruction to the smooth flow of Liver Qi.*

- **Season:** *spring. This is the time of year when new growth bursts forth, the energy moves upwards and outwards and the sap rises.*

- **Climate:** *wind. Just as the wind causes branches of trees to shake, Wind in the body manifests as shaking and tremor. The spring is a time when Liver imbalances are more prone to appear as the spring winds blow.*

LIVER AND GALL BLADDER CHANNELS

Points	Functions	Used to treat
Liv2 Moving Between*	Clears Heat, smooths Liver Qi	Headache, vertigo
Liv3 Great Pouring*	Smooths Liver Qi, strengthens Blood	Headache, high blood pressure, insomnia, painful periods, irritability, depression, pre-menstrual irritability and breast soreness
Liv5 Woodworm Canal	Smooths Liver Qi, transforms DampHeat	Genital herpes, yellow vaginal discharge
Liv8 Curved Spring	Benefits Bladder, clears and cools DampHeat	Vaginal discharge, cystitis, knee problems
Liv13 Camphorwood Gate	Strengthens and regulates Spleen, smooths Liver Qi	Indigestion, vomiting, diarrhoea, constipation, pain at the sides of the upper abdomen
Liv14 Gate of Hope	Smooths Liver Qi, relaxes the chest, transforms DampHeat	Indigestion, pre-menstrual syndrome
GB12 Completion Bone	Dispels Wind, Cold and Heat, calms the mind	Headache
GB20 Wind Pool	Disperses Wind, WindCold and WindHeat, calms Liver Qi	Headache, common cold, rash, dizziness, deafness, pain and stiffness in neck and shoulder
GB21 Shoulder Well*	Spreads Liver Qi, calms Liver Qi	Pain and stiffness in neck and shoulder
GB29 Squatting Bone-hole	Strengthens lower back and hip, dispels Wind, Cold and Heat	Low back pain and pain in hip
GB30 Jumping Circle	Clears the channels	Pain in hip, pain which radiates down back or side of leg
GB34 Yang Mound Spring	Strengthens and regulates Liver Qi, smooths Liver Qi, transforms DampHeat	Headache, constipation, pain and stiffness in knee, sciatica
GB39 Hanging Bell	Regulates Gall Bladder, calms Liver Wind, clears Heat, strengthens bone, helps ears	Migraine, tinnitus, deafness, pain in joints and legs
GB40 Hill Ruins	Smooths Liver Qi, clears channels	Pain in ankle
GB41 Foot Verge of Tears	Regulates Liver Qi, transforms DampHeat	Sciatic pain down side of leg, pre-menstrual breast soreness and distension, painful periods, headache

* Do not use during pregnancy

traditions and Chinese medicine is no different. The associated organ is the Kidney, which is the most important organ in Chinese medicine since it is the root of the yin and yang of the whole body and is where *Jing* (Essence) is stored. Jing is the foundation of our constitution. If the Kidney is weak, the other organs of the body tend to suffer as the source is depleted. If there is long-term illness or a lifestyle which weakens organs, the Kidney will eventually become depleted.

The Kidney is responsible for Water metabolism in general, but the lower parts of the body in particular are controlled by Kidney function. Oedema in the legs and thighs, and swellings, such as seen with cellulite, are a consequence of a depletion of Kidney energy. The Kidney is also related to the function and strength of bones and it generates Marrow which passes up the spinal column to the brain; mental activity, memory and concentration are a result of Kidney function.

The Kidney draws Qi down from the Lung and so helps the Lung to send Qi downwards and outwards. The two organs together are related to normal breathing: imbalances may lead to breathlessness, cough and wheezing.

Disturbances of the Kidney

Weakness of Kidney Qi leads to symptoms of frequent urination, urination at night, low back pain, weak knees, decreased sexual desire, impotence, premature ejaculation, infertility, pallor and tiredness. In severe cases there are cold feelings, water swelling and waking at 4–5am with diarrhoea. Weakness of Kidney Yin (Water) leads to Dryness and Heat within the body, with symptoms of night sweats, increased sexual desire, low back pain, dry throat, constipation with dryness of the stools, tinnitus and deafness.

KIDNEY ASSOCIATIONS

- **Colour:** *black. This is the colour of yin and is therefore associated with the Water element and thus the Kidney. It explains the change of skin colour in sunlight as the yin arises from within the body to meet the yang of the sun in order to balance the energies.*

- **Emotions:** *fears and phobias. In terms of human health, the time of winter is late in life, the time before death. Psychologically, the Kidney is related to the deep unconscious.*

- **Mental associations:** *intellect, intelligence and wisdom, insight and quality of intelligence. Will, ambition and drive also depend upon Kidney function.*

- **Sense organ:** *ear. The ear, of course, is the same shape as the Kidney. Deafness and tinnitus are frequently the result of Kidney imbalances.*

- **Paired organ:** *Urinary Bladder. This receives impure fluids and expels them to the outside as urine.*

- **Taste:** *salty. Excess salty taste will damage the Kidneys. This phenomenon is already familiar in the West, since eating too much salty food can lead to excessive strain on the kidneys and, consequently, high blood pressure.*

- **Time:** *5–7pm. This is the time when Kidney energy is at its peak. Conversely, 5–7am is the time when it is lowest. This is when death is most common and when weakness of the Kidney may manifest.*

- **Season:** *winter. The energy of winter is cold, drawing in and down so that the yang of the body is protected during the cold months of winter.*

- **Climate:** *cold. When I was a child I remember being told not to walk barefoot on a cold floor or I would get a chill in my kidneys; the Kidney channel begins in the sole of the foot (see page 66).*

KIDNEY AND URINARY BLADDER CHANNELS

Points	Functions	Used to treat
K3 Great Ravine	Strengthens Kidney Yin	Low back pain, deafness, insomnia
K6 Shining Sea	Cools Heat, calms Spirit, benefits the throat	Tonsillitis, sore throat, dry cough
K7 Recover Flow	Strengthens Kidney Yang	Low back pain, impotence, vaginal discharge
K10 Yin's Valley	Strengthens Kidneys, clears Heat	Knee pain/swelling, cystitis, vaginal discharge
UB10 Celestial Pillar	Disperses Wind, reduces fever, clears Heat	Headache, stiff and painful neck
UB12 Wind Gate	Regulates Lungs, disperses Wind and Cold	Common cold, fevers, cough
UB13 Lung Transporting Point	Strengthens Lungs, disperses WindCold and WindHeat, transforms Phlegm	Common cold, cough, tiredness, pain and stiffness of neck and upper back
UB15 Heart Transporting Point	Strengthens and regulates Heart, calms Spirit	Anxiety, insomnia, menopausal symptoms
UB17 Diaphragm Transporting Point	Strengthens and regulates Spleen and Blood, cools Heat in the Blood, helps the diaphragm	Anaemia, rash, painful periods, headache, hiccups
UB18 Liver Transporting Point	Smooths Liver Qi, strengthens Liver	Tinnitus and deafness, belching, indigestion
UB19 Gall Bladder Transporting Point	Regulates and transforms DampHeat in Liver and Gall Bladder, clears Liver Heat, helps eyes	Gall stones, insomnia, pain in flanks, red and sore eyes
UB20 Spleen Transporting Point	Strengthens and regulates Spleen and Stomach, transforms Dampness	Indigestion, poor appetite, anxiety, diarrhoea, constipation
UB21 Stomach Transporting Point	Strengthens and regulates Spleen and Stomach, transforms Dampness and DampHeat	Indigestion, poor appetite, belching, nausea, vomiting
UB23 Kidney Transporting Point	Strengthens Kidneys, promotes urination	Low back pain, vaginal discharge, diarrhoea
UB25 Large Intestine Transporting Point	Regulates and moistens Intestines, helps lower back	Haemorrhoids, constipation, diarrhoea, low back pain
UB37 Gate of Abundance	Strengthens lower back, relaxes tendons	Pain in leg, low back pain
UB40 Bend Middle	Dispels Wind, helps lower back and knees	Pain down back of leg, low backache
UB57 Support the Mountain	Regulates Large Intestine	Haemorrhoids, low backache, sciatic pain
UB60 Kunlun Mountains*	Relaxes sinews and muscles, helps lower back	Low backache, sciatic pain down back of leg

* Do not use during pregnancy

CHAPTER THREE

LIFESTYLE
MEDITATION · DIET · DAILY LIFE

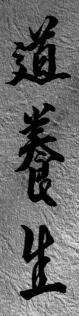

- *Keeping healthy*
- *How your lifestyle affects your health*
- *Simple meditation exercises to practise at home*
- *Applying Chinese dietary principles*

As we discovered in chapter two, in Chinese medicine health is considered to be a balance of Qi and Blood. This is a dynamic process and is dependent upon many factors, one of the most influential of which is our lifestyle. How we live our lives, whether relaxed or stressed, as well as diet and exercise, influences our sense of well-being. However, there is no value in advising everyone to pursue the same level of exercise or the same diet; the key issue, therefore, is what suits each one of us personally.

HOW TO BE HEALTHY

Essentially, the Chinese view of health is that moderation is essential in whatever activity we are involved with. It is the extremes of excess and abstinence which are frequently associated with ill-health. This is the first message of Chinese medicine – relax! There is no value in following an extreme of behaviour in the belief that it is healthy if the result is only stress and tension.

There are a number of factors to consider which influence our health, and these are discussed below (two of these – constitution and climate – have already been introduced in chapter two, but it is important to mention them again here as they have a role to play in how we adjust our lifestyle).

CONSTITUTION

This is the strength of our energy in this life and is, to a large extent, something that we are born with (*see page 22*). Generally, it cannot be easily strengthened, but Qi Gong, meditation and herbs can be effective in this. This is because Qi and Blood are generated by these methods and can then be transformed into Jing. In Chinese medicine, Jing is a fundamental substance inherited from our parents which controls growth, development and fertility. It is governed by long cycles of seven years (for females) and eight years (for males) within the body. Females, for example, attain puberty at around fourteen years of age and menopause at around forty-nine years; males pass through a 'menopausal' time at sixty-four years.

Our constitution is not merely the result of events in this life. In common with beliefs across the whole of Asia and increasingly in the West, it is recognized by Chinese medicine that influences from previous lives have an effect on our current situation, and this includes our health. However, whatever constitution we are born with, we can make the most of it by a healthy and balanced lifestyle.

PRE-EXISTING LIFESTYLE

It is commonly recognized that our lifestyle affects our ability to be healthy. In the West in particular, people live at a fast pace with little time for rest and relaxation. Stress is seen as one of the most powerful things we have to deal with in the modern world; long-term exposure to high stress levels and emotional disturbances has a strong effect on us. Chinese medicine takes the view that it is not necessarily the level of stress that is the problem, though of course this is relevant, but more importantly it is *how* we react to the world we live in.

There are methods which can allow us to live more healthily whatever situation in which we find ourselves. The meditation practices described later in this chapter are very useful in helping us to strengthen ourselves, and Qi Gong (described in chapter four) has a similar effect. Rest and relaxation allow Qi and Blood to be strong, healthy and circulate harmoniously. In this way, ill-health is less likely and we can live life to our full potential. There are many other examples of activities which can damage particular organs: for example, smoking tends to damage Lung energy and leads to Dryness of the Lungs, whereas excessive physical work tends to weaken the lower back and thus the Kidney energy.

CLIMATE

Our external environment influences the level or type of exercise and the diet that is most appropriate. In today's world, the effects of climate are less obvious as we tend not to be in contact with nature so much. People who live in rural areas are much more aware of the effects of the climate on their lives. I remember vividly when I first moved to rural Ireland from London, I went outside without a hat one day when it was cold and windy. Within fifteen minutes I experienced a stabbing headache with a stiff neck. These are the classical symptoms of a WindCold invasion.

Although modern life does separate us from nature, we may still be subject to effects similar to natural climatic factors. An example of this is the use of air-conditioning units, which subject people to draughts and dry air. The basic tenet of Chinese medicine is that climatic factors only gain entrance into the body when there is already some kind of imbalance. If you are energetically strong then you tend not to suffer from invasion of climatic influences. The different climatic factors are listed on page 22 and their association with particular organs is discussed in chapter two (*see pages 31–40*).

SEASONS

The time of year is also important when it comes to our health. As the length of the day, the temperature and the climate change, it is healthy for us to change our level of activity. For instance, in the winter it is important to go to bed early and get up late. In this way, we can be spared the excesses of the harsh weather and be more in tune with the energy of winter (animals, of course, may hibernate at this time). Not living in harmony with the energy of winter affects the Kidneys, leading to tiredness and weakness in the spring. In the summer, it is helpful to get up early and to go to bed later, as yang energy is flourishing at this time and so more activity is appropriate. Not living in harmony with the energy of summer may damage the Heart and lead to fevers in the autumn.

The spring and autumn are intermediate seasons. Here it is beneficial to sleep early and to get up early. Not living in harmony with the energy of spring may damage the Liver and lead to colds in the summer, whereas such activity in the autumn may damage the Lungs and lead to diarrhoea in the winter.

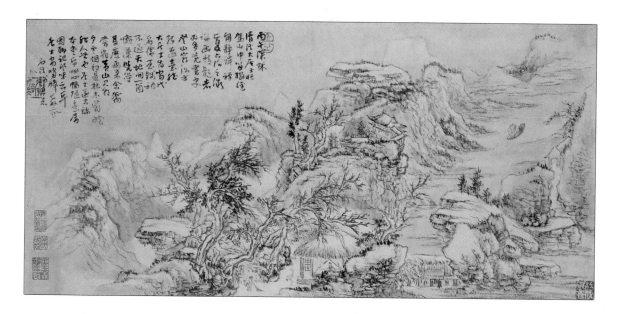

A painting of a winter landscape by Ts'an dated 1666. The season of winter is yin within yin, and to reflect this the landscape and the trees here are depicted in rounded yin forms.

PHYSICAL ACTIVITY

Appropriate levels of exercise are a balance between work/exercise and rest. In the West people tend to overdo most things, and exercise is no exception. The sight of joggers and athletes running to exhaustion, especially in cold weather, is not something that the Chinese would associate with health!

Every morning, in parks and streets all over China, there are literally hundreds of people of all ages performing their daily exercises of Qi Gong and Tai Chi Chuan *(see overleaf)*. These are gentle exercises which help the physical body and generate Qi and Blood.

The Spleen is concerned with muscles, their bulk and their function. Overuse of muscles may weaken the Qi of the Spleen; if the overuse is mainly in one area, such as one arm, there may be obstruction to the flow of Qi. This is commonly seen in conditions

such as tennis elbow, which is overuse of the forearm. Lifting affects the lower back and so may weaken the Qi of the Kidney.

The basic rule about exercise is that if it leads to exhaustion, it depletes the Qi. This is particularly harmful during puberty, especially in girls, where it may result in menstrual problems later in life. Conversely, inadequate exercise tends to lead to obstruction to the flow of Qi which may be associated with Dampness (mucus). This is common in relation to office and computer work, and causes feelings of tiredness, heaviness and lethargy. Gentle forms of exercise which are beneficial in this situation are walking, cycling and swimming.

SEXUAL ACTIVITY

The level of sexual activity which is appropriate for any particular person depends upon the individual, their age, their general level of health and the time of year. Sexual desire is related to the strength of Kidney energy. Sexual fluids such as semen are the outward

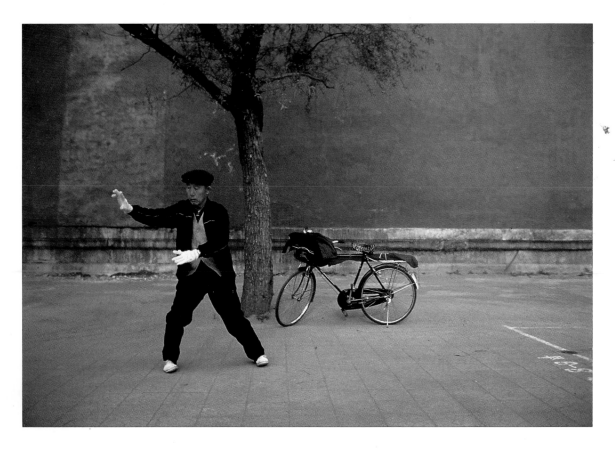

Tai Chi is a common form of exercise in China, and is practised every morning as part of a daily routine. It provides physical benefits, strengthens Qi and calms the mind.

manifestations of Kidney Jing. Since Jing is a fundamental substance related to constitutional strength and longevity, excess sexual activity is considered to be a cause of ill-health because it depletes Kidney Jing. In men, 'excess' means frequent ejaculation. It is more difficult to deplete the Jing of women through sexual activity, although pregnancy and childbirth tend to do this. With this in mind, the Chinese have, over the centuries, developed methods of retaining semen during sexual intercourse so that semen, and hence Jing, is not lost. Such methods belong to the tradition of Qi Gong practice and involve specific physical exercises, breathing control and Qi exercises.

Sexual activity is more depleting if you are intoxicated or tired. It is also important to avoid exposure to cold afterwards. Sexual activity may weaken the Kidney, and this may be the origin of the old wives' tale that excessive masturbation or sexual activity may cause backache, weak knees, poor hearing and a weak brain. Lack of sexual activity may also lead to ill-health, although meditation and Qi Gong exercises can help to transform energies. Ultimately, sexual activity can be part of a spiritual practice where this energy ascends to the Heart, and this is utilized in advanced meditations.

INJURY

Injuries cause localized obstructions to the flow of Qi and Blood. If the injury is slight then Qi is affected, but in more severe cases Blood is involved; symptoms such as pain and swelling are experienced. Obstruction to Blood flow manifests as bruising. Most injuries resolve themselves, but in some cases an internal problem may develop later due to the site of the injury. For example, injury at the point CV17 (*see page 26*) may later lead to cough, wheezing, upper-body swelling and the coughing of blood because of its connection with the energy of the Lungs and Heart. Injury at Sp10 (*see page 26*) may lead to dizziness and blurred vision, as it is an important point in regulating Blood function. Treatment of such injuries should be prompt.

PARASITES AND POISONS

Disease may be caused by taking in poisons or spoiled or uncooked food; numbers of cases in the West have increased in recent years. Travel to tropical countries is also associated with such stomach and bowel disorders.

Parasites such as worms like hot and damp conditions. If Heat and Dampness accumulate in the Intestines, worms will congregate. This is the case in children, where a weak Spleen and Stomach leads to the accumulation of Dampness, and Heat builds up as the flow of Qi is obstructed. Treating the Spleen and Stomach as well as avoiding those foods which lead to the accumulation of Heat and Dampness (*see page 55*) remedies the situation.

INAPPROPRIATE TREATMENT

This is an increasingly common problem, as people have treatment which does not take account of underlying imbalances in Qi and Blood. This is somewhat controversial as conventional Western medicines are frequently placed in this category. The reason is that although they remove the symptoms of disease, they do so by removing Qi or Blood from the body. This leads to a depletion in the energy of the person and is, in any case, not curative as removal of the medicine often leads to a reappearance of the symptoms.

This discussion should not be misunderstood. There are clearly occasions when conventional medicine is necessary, such as for serious disease or in life-threatening situations. However, long-term treatment with powerful chemicals tends to deplete a person's energy. Gentler methods of strengthening or harmonizing may be more appropriate.

Chinese medicines may also be given inappropriately over a long period of time, and I have certainly seen some cases where this has led to disease. For example, ginseng can do this when taken on its own, particularly in people who have Blood weakness as it is heating in its effect. A variety of symptoms may develop, including overheating of the Heart energy with night sweats, hot feelings in the chest, palpitations and anxiety. The important point is that an assessment has to be made of the person's energy, Qi and Blood, and an appropriate treatment given which will lead to a healthy balance.

MENTAL AND EMOTIONAL HEALTH

In the West, it is not unusual to find that people overuse their mental functions. Long working hours, going to bed late, and eating on the move or irregularly all tend to be common. The Qi becomes exhausted, especially the Qi of the Stomach, Spleen and Kidney. There is no time for us to rest and replenish our stores; even at night in cities, constant noise is absorbed and our minds cannot rest during sleep.

One of the most effective methods for strengthening ourselves mentally and emotionally is meditation. If you have a specific emotional or mental symptom, often when it arises it is strong in nature, uncomfortable and interferes with your life. If this is the case, it is because your particular emotion or thought is stronger than you. With techniques of meditation and methods of increasing your energy, you will become stronger and not be overwhelmed by such symptoms. Eventually, they become controllable and will subside.

I would encourage you to consider some of the following meditation practices to improve your health in general and increase your sense of well-being, but you can also strengthen yourself by means of Qi Gong practices, dietary changes and massage. The Qi Gong exercises in chapter four are particularly relevant to the following discussion about meditation.

MEDITATION

Of all the methods available to Chinese medicine this is considered to be the most important aspect. In a Han dynasty work it is stated that it is most important to nourish the spirit, and is only of secondary importance to nourish the body. The spirit should be 'pure and tranquil', and the bones should be 'stable'; this, it is believed, is the foundation of long life. The Tibetans agree and say, 'The mind is King'. It is the innermost aspect of ourselves as human beings, and therefore the most essential but also, perhaps, the most difficult to access. However, it is at the level of the mind that true miracles can occur. These may be in terms of our health, where meditation or visualization exercises can sometimes reverse serious diseases. More often, it leads to an increased level of emotional and mental well-being due to its ability to directly transform negative states of mind.

There are several strands to Chinese medicine, and the two most significant are Taoist and Buddhist influences. The ultimate goal of these two philosophical systems (which some would describe as religions) is enlightenment – the realization of our oneness, of our true nature, of our ability to be limitlessly wise and compassionate (*see also page 20*). Meditation is the method to attain such realizations.

There are several levels at which meditation can be practised. You can practise it purely on a mundane level to attain relaxation and joy. On a more spiritual level, it is possible to practise meditation to attain freedom from suffering and allow your true nature, your 'compassionate heart' to shine forth.

WHAT IS MEDITATION?

Simply, meditation is a state of mind which does not seek to manipulate thoughts and emotions but merely to allow them to settle of their own accord. For some people, this may occur when they are absorbed in some simple task or when they are in a particularly relaxed state of mind. If this is the case with yourself, use this experience when you begin the meditation practices described on page 51. If not, the practice of meditation will allow you to experience such stillness and relaxation. As the thoughts and emotions settle, the natural clarity of the mind is revealed and its natural radiance, which is compassion, is able to emerge.

But what is 'mind'? There are many levels of mind or consciousness; two of these are considered here. The ordinary, judgemental mind is usually the mind of our everyday existence and the one which leads us into all sorts of difficulties and problems. It seeks to see the world in terms of dualities, of good and bad, of attachment and aversion. It is the mind which reacts to situations with anger, irritation, impatience, jealousy and so forth. The innermost level of mind has different terms according to the particular spiritual or religious tradition. This mind can be considered to be sky-like in nature, yet aware, clear, unobstructed and limitless in its wisdom and compassion.

Meditation can be learnt and practised by anyone. The methods described here are simple ways for anyone of any spiritual or religious inclination to allow their mind to calm and to settle. When you first begin to meditate you may notice that your mind seems to become noisier and busier. This shows that the meditation is working because you have started to become aware of the 'internal chatter' which normally goes unnoticed in our busy lives. With time, thoughts settle and emotions are calmed.

MEDITATION POSTURE

The most important thing about meditation posture is that the back should be upright so that the spine is vertical. The back is traditionally said to be like a 'pile of golden coins' or 'straight as an arrow'. There is a natural curve in the lower part of the back so do not strain or sit unnaturally; allow your back to settle in an upright position. The head should be slightly inclined downwards and the gaze softly focused in front (*see overleaf*). The tradition of meditation with which I am familiar teaches that the eyes should be open. This is so that we are not cut off from the world but can integrate all of our experiences. If you find it more comfortable with your eyes closed when you begin, then do so. This is associated with sleep, so if sleepiness or tiredness is a problem, open your eyes slightly to increase your alertness. If your mind becomes overactive, you may find it helpful to lower your gaze.

Sit on a chair or cross-legged on the floor. The important thing is to be comfortable; 'lotus' positions for the legs are not necessary at the beginning of practice. Relax your body and breathing, and release any areas of tension particularly in the neck, jaw and shoulders. The tip of your tongue should touch the roof of your mouth behind the upper teeth. This is to connect the energy flow around your body. Breathe softly and gently through your mouth and nose.

FOCUS OF MEDITATION

There are several things which you can use as a focus during your meditation. Such a focus allows your mind to settle. Eventually, you can 'let go' of the method when your mind is more stable and enters meditation more naturally. The two methods covered here are focusing on the breath and focusing on an object; these are featured in the practices on page 51. The third method is focusing on a mantra. A mantra is defined as that which protects the mind. It is a chanted phrase which is the embodiment of a particular quality. A common mantra in China is *Om Mani Padme Hum*, the Buddhist mantra of compassion. It is also found in Tibetan Buddhism.

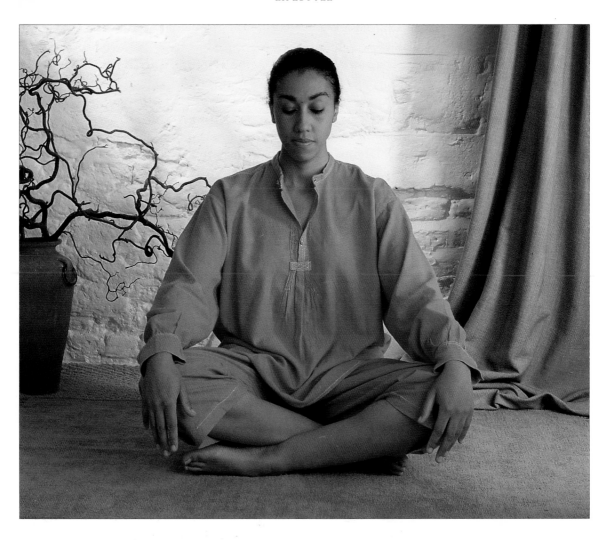

Above. *A typical meditation posture: the back is straight, the head slightly inclined downwards, with the gaze lowered or softly focused ahead, and the whole body is relaxed. Above all, be comfortable.*

Right. *When you first start to practise the breathing relaxation exercise, placing your hands on your upper chest and abdomen will help you ensure that your chest remains still as you breathe. With practice, this will become more natural.*

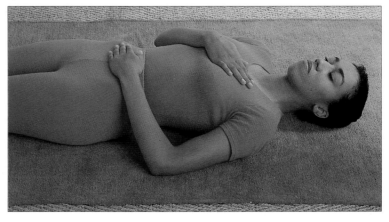

MEDITATION PRACTICES

Breathing relaxation

This practice is a simple method of breathing in a relaxed manner and using the whole of the lungs. It is known as abdominal or diaphragmatic breathing and aids relaxation. Bringing the breath down into the abdomen makes our breathing more efficient and releases deeply held tensions.

Either use the meditation posture described previously or lie down in a warm and comfortable place. As you breathe in, let your abdomen expand and your chest remain still (*see below left*). In this way, the diaphragm moves down, the lungs expand and air is drawn into them. As you breathe out, let your abdomen move in so that air is expelled from your lungs. Continue this practice for several minutes and focus on your breath entering and leaving your body – on your abdomen slowly rising and falling. Gradually, with practice, you will find that your breathing, body and mind become more relaxed.

Focusing on the breath

Adopt the meditation posture and try this exercise which gently focuses on the breath.
• As you breathe in and out, gently become aware of the flow of breath entering and leaving your body.
• As you breathe in, allow your breath to soften and release any areas of tension and discomfort.
• As you breathe out, release this tension.
• As thoughts and emotions arise in your mind, do not follow them or become involved in them – merely watch them rise and fall. Watch them pass like clouds in the sky.

With each in-breath and out-breath you become more and more relaxed. Use your breath as your focus, but do not concentrate on it too much. Direct only part of your attention to your breath and allow your mind to remain relaxed yet alert.

Focusing on an object

This is very similar to the previous practice. You can use any object for your focus, although you should try to find something that you find inspiring. This could be a flower, a beautiful picture, a religious figure, a photograph or painting from nature – whatever connects with you. As you calm your mind, gently focus on the object. Allow your mind to settle and peacefully relax. Whenever you find that you are distracted, gently bring your attention back to the object.

Visualization

Use the meditation posture described previously, and relax your body and mind. You are now going to visualize your body as being healthy and whole. As you breathe in, imagine breathing in white light. This is healing and cooling and energizing. Each time you breathe in, you breathe in more and more healing light. Concentrate on areas of tension or discomfort in particular; if you have a specific disease or illness, you can pay special attention to it, sending healing light to that area. As you breathe out, visualize all tension, discomfort and problems leaving your body as dark smoke. Each breath causes more dark smoke to leave you.

Continue this practice for as long as you can, until your whole body has been filled by white light and is totally healed. All problems have been removed and your body is now shining with white, healing and energizing light. There are two recommendations that make this practice particularly powerful:
• Make sure that when you finish the practice, you have a sense that all problems have been removed. Do not leave a little bit over until the next time.
• Practise daily for maximum benefit.

MEDITATION IN YOUR LIFE

All the teachers and meditation masters agree that regular practice produces the greatest results. With meditation and visualization for a specific health problem, the degree of recovery is directly related to the amount of time spent in meditation.

However, when we begin to practise it can be immensely difficult to find the time. We lead busy lives with many distractions and meditation can be the last thing we come to, even though we may know of its benefits. Practise meditation each day for an amount of time that is comfortable for you. There is no set time that you should practise for: to begin with, five or ten minutes may be enough. It is better to start with a short, manageable period, than to fail at a longer period of time. The time of day when you practise should also be to suit you, although you may find that practising in the morning is more helpful because this is when our energy is fresher and stronger. The traditional time for meditation or Qi Gong is when the sun is rising.

Consider the environment of your meditation. Choose a favourite place in your house or in the garden; meditating outdoors in direct contact with nature can be very inspiring and can greatly benefit practice. Perhaps have a small area in your house or bedroom which is devoted to meditation. Consider using flowers, a beautiful picture, lighting incense or having an inspiring object in your meditation area: meditation provides an inspiring environment for your mind – it can be helped by providing such an environment in your physical surroundings. The main point here is that you are creating a space in which your meditation can occur, and this is reflected in a space within your mind. Thus, thoughts and emotions settle allowing your inner clarity to arise.

Seeking further guidance

The exercises in this book can be applied easily and simply. With practice you will notice definite changes. However, you may reach a stage where you need further guidance or help in understanding your experiences in meditation; this is the time to find a teacher. You should only receive guidance when you are satisfied that a teacher can give you what you need; make an assessment of their qualifications and training, and discuss their particular tradition of meditation and its origins with them (see chapter eight for more advice on choosing a teacher). You may also find it helpful to refer to 'The Tibetan Book of Living and Dying', which is full of practical advice on meditation and the mind (see page 157).

DIET AND HEALTH

The preparation of food for ourselves and our loved ones is one of the oldest traditions of humankind. It is intimately linked with our health and how we interrelate with our relatives and friends. How food is prepared, cooked and eaten has an important role to play in health; this is recognized by Chinese medicine, where it is not only the type of food which is seen to be important but also its energy. This is a consequence of the view that Qi underlies all existence. Therefore, the particular Qi of each food is a key factor as well as its preparation and cooking, both of which can change this energy. Today, we also have to take into account factors such as processing and agricultural methods.

In China itself, people may be given prescriptions by a doctor for a certain food or meal which they then take to an adjoining restaurant. The restaurant prepares the meal in the way specified by the prescription and it is then eaten purely with the purpose of improving health. There is no such 'health-food' restaurant in the West, but this shows the relationship that the Chinese believe exists between our diet and our health. Treating illness by means of diet has a long history in Chinese medicine, as can be seen by its inclusion in the 'Yellow Emperor's Inner Classic' (*Huangdi Neijing*), written around 300 BC (*see page 11*).

Such dietary therapy is merely one example of how knowledge of energy can be used to balance a person's Qi and Blood. Chinese medicine allows us to determine the condition of our own energy and then gives us the tools by which we can balance it or ensure that it remains in balance. Chinese medicine seeks to cool what is hot and warm what is cold. If we are constitutionally cold, it is helpful to eat foods which are warm in nature and have been warmed in their preparation. If we are constitutionally hot, it is helpful to eat foods which are cooling. You will have noticed that the symptoms of specific imbalances listed in chapter two reveal symptoms of coldness or heat. In such cases, foods would be suggested to attain a balance.

FOOD ENERGIES

In the West, we tend to concentrate on a particular food and how much of it we eat. There are foods which are considered harmful and therefore should be avoided. Other foods are considered to be healthy and are advised to be eaten in large quantities. If we consider the energetic qualities of food, it can be seen that it is not the amount of food which is the prime factor to be taken into consideration. It is the ways in which foods are combined or how they are cooked which are important. A balance of foods and tastes is the healthiest way to approach diet; moderation in all things sums up the Chinese approach to diet.

The energies of foods were determined by masters of meditation and Qi Gong who experienced the effect of foods on their own energy. These methods were also used to determine energies of herbs. The distinction between a herb and a food is a somewhat artificial one. Herbs may be used as foods in some situations and foods used as herbs in others. What is important is to consider our own energies and how we can use herbs and foods to ensure they are balanced.

Most of us already take food energies into account, although we may not think in those terms. Eating lamb with rosemary, beef with horseradish sauce, duck with orange, soybean curd (tofu) with fresh ginger are all examples of combining foods whose qualities complement one another. There are several qualities of food which are taken into consideration:

• Qi: cold, cool, neutral, warm, hot.
• Taste: sweet, spicy (pungent), sour, bitter, salty, aromatic, bland.
• The organ that is influenced.

The chart overleaf shows the different tastes and their effects; bland is a category of taste which is not ascribed to any particular organ, and so it is not featured in the chart. Examples of foods with different energies are given on page 55 (please note that foods can sometimes have more than one function: for example, beef nourishes Yin and Blood and also warms Yang and Qi).

TASTES AND THEIR EFFECTS

Taste	Organ affected	Effect	Effect of excess	Example
Sweet	Spleen	Strengthening, relieves pain	Formation of Dampness and Phlegm, which obstruct flow of Qi and lead to Heat	Honey, sugar
Spicy	Lungs	Helps circulation of Qi and Blood	Overstimulating, damages Qi and Blood	Black pepper, chilli, cayenne
Sour	Liver	Stops sweating, diarrhoea	Retention of water	Vinegar, lemon
Bitter	Heart	Relieves fever, stops cough and wheeze, purgative	Weakens the Qi, drying	Dandelion, asparagus
Salty	Kidneys	Softens and disperses hard lumps	Obstructs flow of Blood	Seaweed, salt
Aromatic	Spleen	Awakens Spleen Qi, relieves Dampness	Drying	Cardamom

Special recommendations

With regard to certain sections of the population, namely young children, pregnant women and the elderly, there are certain foods that are beneficial, and some that should be avoided altogether. The advice below offers general guidance on diet in each case.

Babies and young children

Children grow rapidly, and so need good sources of protein such as meat, eggs or pulses together with plenty of vegetables. You should follow the advice in the box opposite to ensure that your child has a generally healthy diet.

Pregnant women

If you are pregnant, you should avoid foods of hot energy and those with a spicy (pungent) taste, such as chillies, cinnamon and wines. These may damage the body fluids

A HEALTHY DIET FOR BABIES AND INFANTS

Do:
- *Breast-feed if possible, and when relaxed.*
- *Start mixed feeding at six months and not before three months. Your baby will let you know when to start solids.*
- *Begin solid food by dry-toasting rice in a hot pan until lightly browned. Add water and cook.*
- *Feed well-cooked grains and warmly cooked vegetables, which are the mainstay of a healthy diet.*

Don't:
- *Breast-feed directly after hard work or sexual intercourse.*
- *Feed raw foods, including raw fruit.*
- *Introduce more than one new food per day (allow your child to become accustomed to the new taste).*
- *Feed junk food, processed food or tinned food.*
- *Feed cold, greasy and excessively sweet tastes (this means sugar and foods to which sugar has been added).*

FOOD ENERGY

Energy/Function	Foods
Cold	Banana, crab, dandelion, grapefruit, kelp, mango, salt, seaweed, sprouted mung bean, tea, tomato, water chestnut, watermelon, white pepper
Cool	Apple, aubergine (eggplant), barley, buckwheat, chard, cucumber, lettuce, marjoram, millet, mung bean, mushroom (button), orange (mandarin), pear, peppermint, radish, soybean curd (tofu), spinach, tangerine, watercress, wheat
Neutral	Aduki bean, apricot, beef, beetroot, broad bean, cabbage, carrot, celery, corn, crab-apple, duck, egg (chicken), fig, grape, green bean, herring, honey, kidney bean, liquorice, milk (cow), olive, pineapple, pea, peanut, plum, pork, potato, pumpkin, rice, rye, sardine, turnip, yam
Warm	Almond, anchovy, asparagus, basil, cardamom, cherry, chestnut, chicken, chives, cinnamon bark (*Gui Pi*), coconut, coffee, coriander, date, dill seed, fenugreek, fennel seed, garlic, ginger (fresh), lamb, leek, lychee, malt, maltose, mussel, mutton, nutmeg, onion, orange peel, peach, plum (black Chinese), quince, raspberry, rosemary, shrimp, squash, strawberry, sunflower seed, sweet potato, tobacco, vinegar, walnut, wine
Hot	Black pepper, cayenne, chilli, cinnamon bark (*Rou Gui*), ginger (dried), paprika, trout
Nourishes Yin and Blood	Apple, apricot, asparagus, beans (aduki, green, kidney), beef, beetroot, cheese, clam, crab, dandelion, date, duck, egg, grape, honey, leaf greens, liver, malt, mango, milk, nettle, oyster, parsley, pea, pear, pineapple, pork, rabbit, sardine, spinach, sweet rice, soybean curd (tofu), tomato, watercress, watermelon, yam
Warms Yang and Qi	Basil, beef, cherry, chestnut, chicken, chive, clove, coconut, date, dill, fennel seed, garlic, ginger, grape, ham, kidney, lamb, lentil, lobster, mackerel, molasses, mushroom (shiitake), nutmeg, oats, potato, rabbit, raspberry, rosemary, sage, shrimp, soybean curd (tofu), squash, sweet potato, thyme, walnut, yam
Creates Dampness	Beer, banana, dairy foods (goat's milk and cheese is preferable to cow's), greasy food in general, meats (especially greasy ones), orange juice, tofu (soybean curd), wheat (gluten, which is sticky), white sugar, yeast
Resolves Dampness	Alfalfa, barley, beans (aduki, kidney), celery, garlic, lemon, onion, parsley, pumpkin, radish, rye, turnip
Smooths the Flow of Qi	Basil, caraway, cardamom, carrot, cayenne, chive, clove, coriander, dill seed, garlic, marjoram, orange and tangerine peel, radish, turmeric

and thereby affect the foetus. It is fairly common for food cravings to be experienced during pregnancy. Eat a small amount of what you are craving: if the craving disappears, it came from the baby and is now satisfied. If it does not disappear, it is due to an imbalance in your energy and continuing to eat that food may actually prolong the problem. It is advisable to seek professional help to rectify the imbalance.

The elderly

It is particularly beneficial for elderly people to eat dairy products, eggs, vegetables, sesame, walnut and yam. Our bodies become drier with age as our Yin (Water) becomes depleted. The Yang (Fire) therefore tends to become overactive and lead to problems such as high blood pressure. The foods listed above are particularly beneficial as they nourish the Yin. Other foods which can be of benefit are those which create Dampness (*see page 55*), since these increase the fluids in the body.

CHINESE DIETARY PRINCIPLES

The main organs which deal with food are the Stomach and the Spleen. They are responsible for transforming food into Qi and fluid and then transporting the Qi and fluid to other organs. Their healthy functioning is essential if we are to benefit from the food we eat. Caring for the energy of our Spleen and Stomach ensures a healthy and long life, and there are certain principles that can be applied to everyone.

What to eat

As the Stomach is likened to a cooking pot heated by the Qi of the Spleen in Chinese medicine, if you eat warm, lightly cooked food your own energy will not need to 'cook' the food. Eating cold and raw food is similar to building a fire in your living room and then pouring cold water on it! There are, however, occasions where cold food is appropriate, such as in hot climates or for specific health reasons. This is considered similar to using water on a fire which is out of control and threatening to burn the house down or giving off poisonous fumes.

Eat food which is as pure and 'energetic' as possible. Food is of poorer quality when grown on land which has been exposed to artificial fertilizers, pesticides and herbicides. Food which has been pre-cooked, processed and generally denatured has also had its Qi processed. It is preferable to eat food which has been grown organically, picked that day or is as fresh as possible and then cooked; food which has been cooked over twenty-four hours previously is known as 'wrecked' food. Eating foods which grow in your locality is one way to ensure that they are relatively fresh. In these days of supermarkets and hypermarkets, most of our food travels thousands of kilometres to arrive at the shops. In the West, principles of agriculture such as organic farming and permaculture are now providing people with fresh healthy food.

Most foods can be eaten in moderation, but there are certain foods which it is helpful to avoid or at least greatly restrict, particularly if you have a specific health problem. These are mainly items which have a strong energy or are difficult to digest, such as coffee, alcohol, bleached grains (white rice, white flour), white sugar and salt.

Try to use honey in your food instead of sugar, as it still has a moderate sweet taste and is warm in nature; it may, however, lead to Dampness (mucus) if taken in excess. White sugar is refined and of strong taste, and leads to a weakening of the Spleen and Stomach Qi, whereas brown sugar is warming and gently strengthening.

Meat

Meat is fine to eat, but white meat is easier to digest because it is less greasy. Red meat is warming in nature and is good to eat in a cold winter. If you do eat meat, use it like a medicine, perhaps in a stew with a small amount of meat and plenty of vegetables. In this way you will benefit from the warm energy of the meat without weakening the digestion by overloading it. Pork is cold in nature, which explains why it often causes digestive upsets such as diarrhoea; it cools the Qi of the Spleen and Stomach. If you do eat pork, cook it with herbs which are warming, such as ginger, cardamom and cloves.

Fruit

Fruit is generally good to eat, although it is preferable for it to be cooked in a cold climate. Baked or stewed fruit with ginger and cinnamon is warm in energy and helps to support the Qi of the Spleen and Stomach. Tropical fruits are cold and cool the energy much more, so are more appropriate for tropical climates or hot summer days. For instance, eating pineapple or melon in a cold country on a winter's day is an example of not considering both the energy of the climate and the energy of the food.

Individual requirements

You need to consider your own particular situation. A manual worker who is outside in cold weather, for example, needs to eat more food of a warming nature. A person with a tendency to Liver Qi stagnation will need to eat more foods which smooth the flow of Qi. If you have a weakness of Blood, eat more of the foods which nourish Blood. If we can develop an awareness of our own health, we are in the best position to know what is best for us. This is as true for food as it is for exercise, relaxation, work and even medical care.

Climates

In cold climates people generally have problems with Qi as it has to work harder to warm the body. It is important, therefore, to protect and strengthen the Qi in such environments by eating warm food. Warm food means food which is lightly cooked, such as stir-fried or quickly steamed. In this way, vegetables will be hot yet crunchy and full of goodness, and meat (thinly sliced) will cook through very quickly. Also, try to cook food which looks inviting and stimulates the taste. Chinese cooking at its best is an excellent example of combinations of energies, tastes and colours which nourish us even before we eat. Mixing foods with different energies also changes the effect of the food. For example, soybean curd (tofu) is cold in nature; cooking it with ginger and garlic will make it warmer.

In a hot climate, it is appropriate to eat cooling foods such as tropical fruits and some raw food. However, even here we have to protect the energy of the Spleen. In hot climates, people generally have problems with Blood as this has to work harder to cool the body. People tend to overheat and there may be a build up of toxins. Opening the pores and causing a sweat is a method of cooling and detoxifying. Foods which are spicy (pungent) in nature, such as chillies, do this by causing the Lungs to open the energy at the exterior of the body. Eating such foods in a cold climate would leave the body open to cold passing deep into the body through the open pores. Remember to tailor your diet to how you feel and be in tune with the climatic factors which are prevalent at the time.

When to eat

The amount of food that is eaten and the time of day should also be taken into account. The best time to eat a large meal is the morning. The time of the Spleen and Stomach is 7–11am; this is when the energy of these organs is full and flourishing, so it is appropriate to eat a large meal. This is the basis of the old adage, 'Breakfast like a king, lunch like a prince and supper like a pauper'. The Stomach and Spleen need to rest in the evening and during the night, so it is best not to eat too large an evening meal and to try not to eat after about 7pm if possible.

How to eat

Irregular eating, skipping meals and eating whilst distracted all tend to deplete the Qi of the Stomach and Spleen. Watching the television whilst eating means that the Qi and Blood are drawn up to the eyes and a strain is put on the Liver. The Stomach cannot then 'concentrate' on dealing with food. Eating in a relaxed manner with the family in a calm environment is an inherently healthy occupation and will support the energy of the Spleen and Stomach.

Vegetarianism

Vegetarianism has a strong following in the Orient and has developed in the West in recent years. As meat is generally warm in energy, care has to be taken in a cold, damp climate if none is eaten. It may also be helpful to think of other ways of obtaining Qi, such as Qi Gong or meditation, to supplement your diet. Eating a pulse (bean or lentil), grain and nut at the same meal at least once a day is the best way to ensure that sufficient protein is eaten. Also, use food of warming energy such as ginger, cardamom, garlic and cinnamon.

EFFECTS OF COOKING

It is possible to overcook food – for example, the vegetables I ate as a child were boiled for half an hour – and when this happens it destroys their energy. Cooking traditions differ around the world; the French have several sayings about English cooking. They say the English are very cruel to lamb because they kill it twice, once by the butcher and again when it is cooked; they also say that the English only know three vegetables, and two of those are cabbage! This may be a generalized (and inaccurate!) viewpoint, but it does demonstrate the fact that different methods of cooking predominate in different countries. Whatever country you live in, the important thing is that combinations of tastes and foods (*see pages 54 and 55*) ensure that the food is healthy and is directed at particular organs.

Different methods

The way in which food is cooked also affects the energy of food. The methods listed in the box below give an idea of just how our health is affected by ways of cooking.

COOKING METHODS

- **Baking:** *baking in the traditional way in a slow oven tends to help Spleen energy.*
- **Steaming:** *this results in moister food which benefits the Lungs.*
- **Stewing, stir-frying:** *both of these methods are warming in their effect.*
- **Frying, roasting, barbecuing:** *these increase the energy of food and so are more appropriate in a colder climate in the winter (despite the fact that food is usually only barbecued in the summer!).*
- **Microwaving:** *this creates a strong form of energy which is Yang in nature. It disperses the Qi of the food and dries fluids. Long-term ingestion of microwaved food, therefore, leads to a weakening of Spleen and Stomach Qi as well as Dryness in the body which may manifest as Heat.*

A HEALTHY DIET

The diet shown below is considered to be generally healthy and follows the principles of Chinese medicine. Make allowances for climate, time of year and individual condition.

A HEALTHY DIET

- *Eat regularly three times daily.*
- *Eat mainly warm food. This is essential in a cool, temperate climate.*
- *Eat fresh food preferably organically grown.*
- *Eat food grown in season in your locality.*
- *Eat slowly in a relaxed atmosphere.*
- *Use honey and dried fruit in moderation as natural sweeteners.*
- *Eat well-cooked grains.*
- *Eat porridge for breakfast, either with oats or rice (see page 60 for rice porridge).*
- *Eat soups, stews and casseroles. Red meat is fine in moderation, particularly in a cold climate.*
- *Drink herbal teas to aid the digestion, such as fennel, ginger and camomile. Mint tea is helpful after a meal, particularly in a warm climate.*
- *Eat plenty of fresh vegetables and fruit. Fruit needs to be cooked in a cold climate; add ginger and cinnamon.*

Avoid:
- *Excess intake of coffee, alcohol, chocolate and strong stimulants (it is better to avoid these altogether if there is any degree of ill-health).*
- *Processed foods (food in tins or packets, or those with additives).*
- *Bleached grains, white sugar and added salt.*

Recipes

In China, the basic principles that I have introduced in this book are widely understood and most people apply them to their daily diet. Therefore, they adjust their diet to strengthen Qi, nourish Blood and the like as necessary. In general, the foods listed on page 55 can be easily incorporated into your diet to achieve the desired end result. For example, if you wish to nourish Blood eat foods from those listed; use them in soups, or create meals containing more of those kinds of food. At the same time, do not miss out on other foods as you are trying to achieve a balance of Qi and Blood. You should never concentrate on only one type of food to the exclusion of others.

The recipes given here for vegetable soup and rice porridge are basic staples which are highly versatile and can be easily adapted for different effects. They demonstrate how foods and herbs of different energies can be combined, and show that in certain situations herbs can be considered to be food, and vice versa. When cooking, do not use aluminium pans; cook in stainless steel, glass or cast iron pans. Also, you should always try to use home-grown or organic produce. Never use a microwave as this disperses the Qi and dries the fluids – this is not the healthy result you are trying to achieve!

For conversions of weights and measures, please see page 113.

VEGETABLE SOUP

A tradition in China is to make soups with ingredients which may be altered to suit different situations. I have done this here using vegetable soup as a base.

INGREDIENTS
1 tablespoon sesame oil (or good quality olive oil)
1 onion, peeled and chopped
15 g peeled and grated fresh root ginger
4 small potatoes, 1 carrot, 1 parsnip
4 cups of water

METHOD

Heat a pan, pour in the oil and add the onion and ginger. Fry briefly, then add the other ingredients, chopped into small pieces, and stir-fry for a couple of minutes. Add the water and bring to the boil. Simmer for thirty minutes. Add chopped parsley and a pinch of salt and ground black pepper to taste.

To strengthen the Qi and aid digestion
EXTRA INGREDIENTS
10 g ginseng (Ren Shen)
10 g yellow milk-vetch root (Huang Qi)
3 g citrus peel (Chen Pi)
6 g hoelen (Fu Ling)
6 g cardamom (Sha Ren)
2 cups of water

METHOD

Prepare vegetable soup as above. Place all the extra ingredients into a separate pan with the water, boil and then simmer until the liquid has reduced to 1 cup. Add this herbal liquid to the soup five minutes before it is cooked.

To strengthen the Blood
EXTRA INGREDIENTS
10 g Chinese angelica (Dang Gui)
15 g wolfberry (Gou Qi Zi)
2 cups of water

METHOD

Prepare vegetable soup as above. In a separate pan, boil up the extra ingredients in the water and simmer until the liquid has reduced to 1 cup. Add this herbal liquid to the soup five minutes before it is cooked.

RICE PORRIDGE
There are many types of rice. Brown rice is fine to use, but it can be difficult to digest for people with some weakness of the digestive system (if this applies to you, refer to *Indigestion* on page 138 for remedies to strengthen the digestion or eat vegetable soup with the added ingredients to strengthen Qi and aid digestion). Brown rice does not 'fluff up' like white rice and takes longer to cook with more water. Unpolished white rice is also fine to use. Try to avoid the polished rice which is available in packets and bags as this has had essential vitamins and minerals removed. It is important that rice is well-cooked, so test it before eating by making sure that it is soft: squeeze a grain of rice between your thumb and forefinger — it is still uncooked if there is a thickened consistency in the centre. The recipes given here make enough for two people.

INGREDIENTS
100 g brown rice and 3 cups of water
or
*100 g unpolished white rice/basmati rice
and 1 cup of water*

METHOD

For brown rice porridge, soak the rice in the water for one hour (it is easiest to do this in the pan in which you are going to cook it). Place the pan on a stove, bring to the boil and simmer for up to two hours until soft. For white rice porridge, put the rice and water in a pan, bring to the boil and simmer for thirty minutes (you can also use half sticky or glutinous rice and half short-grain rice for this method).

The amount of water you use will determine the thickness of the final result. You can keep the rice porridge and reheat it later; add water as necessary, as it tends to thicken with standing.

Additions

Rice porridge may be eaten on its own for breakfast or used as a base to which other foods may be added, depending upon the situation. I would encourage you to be creative with your rice porridge; the chart below shows how the addition of different foods has different effect within the body.

RICE PORRIDGE ADDITIONS	
Addition	Effect
Brown sugar or honey with sliced fresh root ginger	Strengthens Spleen and Qi
Honey and milk	Nourishes Spleen and Stomach
Green leafy vegetables, sliced fresh root ginger and finely chopped lamb's liver (optional)	Nourishes Blood
Walnuts, chestnuts and finely chopped lamb's kidneys (optional)	Strengthens Kidney
Purslane	Removes Dampness and Heat
Mung beans	Cools in hot weather

A HEALTHIER LIFESTYLE

In this chapter you will have discovered just some of the methods available to Chinese medicine for maximizing health. Prevention is always better than cure and these methods will help you to stay healthy.

In today's world, one of the most beneficial adjustments we can make to our lifestyle is to learn ways of strengthening ourselves psychologically, so that we can cope better with the ever-increasing pace of life. Meditation is an excellent means by which we can do this, as it is frequently our *reactions* to situations, rather than the actual situations themselves, which cause us discomfort. The exercises described on page 51 can be practised by anyone, and with time you will soon experience the benefits of a calm mind and a relaxed body.

With an understanding of Qi and the organs in the body, it is possible to choose food that is appropriate for your particular situation, the climate in which you live and the time of year. Similar ideas are also discussed in chapter six in relation to herbs. There is a fine dividing line between food and herbs: in some circumstances a food will be used for its medicinal effects, and in others a herb will be used as a nourishing food (as you will have seen in the recipes given above, food and herbs can be mixed to help our Qi and Blood). Make sure that you always eat a healthy balance of foods; consider eating more foods which will help your individual health (*see page 55*). Above all, relax. Eating with other people in a harmonious atmosphere is an inherently healthy occupation.

QI GONG

气
功

Qi Gong is a cornerstone of Chinese medicine. It is a basic resource for maintaining your health and well-being, recovering your health when it declines, and developing heightened levels of functioning and 'aliveness'. Whilst other aspects of Chinese medicine are becoming generally established and more widespread in the West, Qi Gong is something that is less well-known; this is set to change as more and more people hear of the benefits it brings.

WHAT IS QI GONG?

You are already familiar with the word 'Qi'; 'Gong' will be less familiar. As with many other Chinese words, there is no exact translation. The original word is open to different interpretations; the one I prefer is 'cultivating', but it can also be translated as 'working with', 'developing' or 'concentrated effort over time'. Essentially, 'Gong' means developing a skill or ability through focused and concentrated effort.

The distinguishing characteristic of Qi Gong, and meditation, is that you do it *yourself*, although there are occasions when a Qi Gong practitioner transmits their energy to another person or even a group. Other treatment methods of Chinese medicine such as herbs and massage address the Qi, but they are external to the individual – *done* to the body.

Qi Gong is a series of exercises (practices) using postures, movement sequences, breathing patterns, meditation and the mind. Like meditation, it is called a 'practice' as it is something we practise, preferably daily, to benefit from its effects. There are hundreds of different styles, schools and traditions of Qi Gong: Taoist, Buddhist, Confucian, Tibetan … in fact, any system for working with energy could be called Qi Gong.

HISTORY

Qi Gong has a long history which spans the whole of recorded culture in China. A carved cylinder from 380 BC and a recently unearthed silk scroll dating back to 168 BC (*see overleaf*) clearly show figures performing exercises, and early doctors professed the effectiveness of doing Qi Gong as preventive medicine. The body of knowledge of Qi Gong accumulated through the ages; however, it was long held in secrecy because of its power, but, as the foundation of a culture, it seeped out and permeated the common consciousness.

Qi Gong practice entered into martial arts training. When the famous Buddhist monk, Bodhidharma, travelled to China, his message was not well received by the Emperor, and he retreated to the Shaolin temple. He observed that the monks were sickly looking

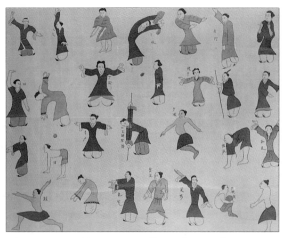

The Daoyin Tu: drawings on silk found at Tomb no. 3, Mawangdui, Changsha, China. The tomb dates to 168 BC.

Marrow Washing', which uses Qi to cleanse and purify the bone marrow, thereby cleansing the Blood, and 'Iron-Shirt' Qi Gong, which 'packs' the fibrous tissue around each muscle with Qi, giving increased strength, resilience and power (an 'iron shirt').

At the beginning of this century, the traditional arts were ignored in the rush to modernize the country and adopt Western technology and science. After the Communists took control in 1949, many of the old practices were reintroduced. During the Cultural Revolution these were discredited and considered counter-revolutionary; this was when Qi Gong spread to the West, as many masters fled from China. Qi Gong teachers can now be found all over the world, and in recent years it has again become recognized for what it is and the benefits which flow from its use.

and unfit, so over a ten-year period he devised Qi Gong practices designed to strengthen the body. These became known as 'Bone-

THE PURPOSE OF QI GONG PRACTICE

Qi Gong addresses one of our most fundamental aspects – our energy. It has many applications and there are many reasons for its practice: fitness, sports, martial arts, health and healing, sexuality, anti-ageing and longevity, well-being, heightened abilities, spirituality and even 'immortality training'. Each of these has its own special and unique forms; as you become more experienced you can progress towards the spiritual practices.

When first beginning to practise Qi Gong, you may have little idea of what your energy is or what it feels like. Qi Gong is not easily translatable into words – you just have to do it, and *feel* the results. Try to describe and define your energy using metaphors for internal sensations, such as colour, temperature, volume and texture. Trust your experience and allow these sensations to cohere into specific images and descriptions. Remember these.

There is a particular state that you may experience during practice: 'The Qi Gong State'. You will begin to learn what it feels like mentally, emotionally and physically. It is a state of attention and awareness of your energy system in which you are able to notice the subtleties and differences of sensation, a state of inner awareness, of quiescence, of quietness.

In the West, with the emphasis on the individual, we tend to focus on *who* we are – our feelings and thoughts (the subjective aspect of ourselves). Qi Gong places our attention on the *objective* aspect of ourselves, of which we are usually unaware; it helps us to focus on *what* we are and *how* we function. If we put our energy system into a correctly functioning state, then we automatically put our feelings and our 'state of being' into correct order.

NATURAL QI GONG

Qi Gong is natural; you already do it every day. It can be described by such terms as resting or recharging. There are certain actions and movements that unconsciously bring us back into balance. These are actions that we all do and are all familiar with (see box below). We bring energy to places where it is deficient and disperse it from places where it is too congested.

NATURAL QI GONG ACTIONS

- *Rubbing your forehead when your have a headache.*
- *Holding your hands over your stomach after eating.*
- *Rubbing your eyes when you are tired.*
- *Stamping your feet when they are cold.*
- *Rubbing your hands together to generate warmth.*
- *Shouting, laughing, singing, weeping, groaning.*

If you learn more about your energy system and Qi Gong, and pay attention to what you are doing and how you are doing it, you will be able to work with your energy and have it under your conscious control rather than being controlled or limited by it.

WALKING

Walking is something that every mobile person does; indeed, for some people it is their primary form of exercise. Walking not only activates the six major channels of the legs, but also utilizes point K1 in the sole of the foot (see page 66) in a significant way, drawing earth energy into you with every step. You can do this consciously and increase your energy intake by bringing your attention to this point as you walk.

PHYSICAL EXERCISE

All physical exercises have an energy component. Although movements are usually done for the physical benefits to muscles and tissue, there is also an unconscious 'energy' reason why they are performed. For instance, athletes do Hard Qi Gong – repetitive actions under force – to develop power and strength, and aerobics stimulates the whole energy system. Dance is a way to activate and stimulate the Qi, and can generate all manner of internal responses, depending on the type of dance.

EXCHANGING ENERGY

Any contact between people involves energy and its exchange; Qi Gong helps us to become aware of our energy. There are basically four levels of exchange, and these are shown below.

LEVELS OF EXCHANGE

i) **Being in a person's energy field** *When your own energy field is directly within that of another person (the field extends about 1 metre, 3–4 feet, from the body), you will have an effect on them, and vice versa.*

ii) **Touching** *Touching someone involves direct physical contact along with a conscious intention. Through this contact you discharge and transmit energy which corresponds to your intention.*

iii) **Hugging** *Hugging someone brings your major internal energy centres – 'Cauldrons' in Chinese medicine, but more familiar to most as 'chakras' – into direct alignment so that exchanges of energy take place.*

iv) **Sex** *This involves a deep level of exchange, wherein yin and yang energies are interchanged between people, ideally complementing and balancing each person's energy.*

THE MAJOR QI GONG POINTS

There are many energy points used in massage and acupuncture. In Qi Gong there are only a small number: these are major energy centres. A knowledge and understanding of these is essential in order to practise. You will find it helpful to memorize their names and locations; the Chinese names have also been given here, as these are the names commonly referred to in Qi Gong

practice. These points are shown below.

The tip of the tongue and the roof of the mouth are also important areas. The tip of the tongue, as in meditation, rests on the roof of the mouth behind the upper teeth. This connects the two major channels which circulate up the back and down the front of the body (the Governor Vessel and the Conception Vessel).

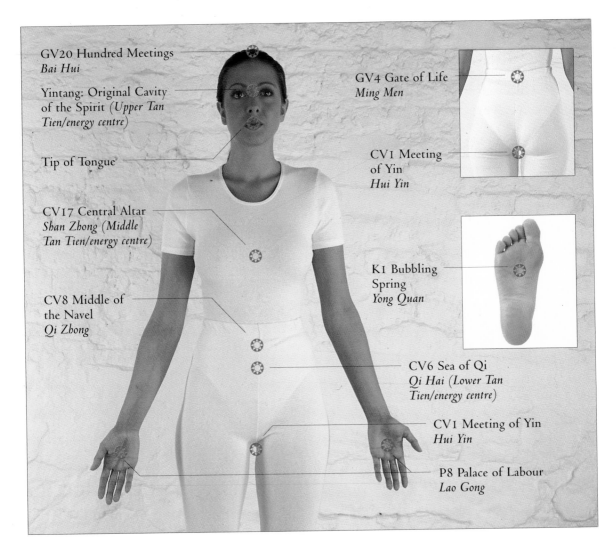

GV20 Hundred Meetings
Bai Hui

Yintang: Original Cavity
of the Spirit (*Upper Tan
Tien/energy centre*)

Tip of Tongue

CV17 Central Altar
Shan Zhong (*Middle
Tan Tien/energy centre*)

CV8 Middle of
the Navel
Qi Zhong

GV4 Gate of Life
Ming Men

CV1 Meeting
of Yin
Hui Yin

K1 Bubbling
Spring
Yong Quan

CV6 Sea of Qi
Qi Hai (Lower Tan
Tien/energy centre)

CV1 Meeting of Yin
Hui Yin

P8 Palace of Labour
Lao Gong

GUIDELINES FOR PRACTICE

The following practices can be performed by anyone in average health, and have been selected and designed to give you an experience of different kinds of practice; all help to develop your overall state of health, and give you a sample of how developing your energy through Qi Gong feels. Follow the instructions generally; try the practices slowly until you have learnt how to do them, then do them in your own way, at your own pace, whenever you need to (see guidelines right).

Find your median point — the state of stillness, of 'centre' in yourself. Learn how to put yourself back into neutral — to push your 'reset button', de-stress and clear yourself. With practice you will learn how to cleanse, generate, increase, accumulate, purify, refine, store and preserve your energy. As you become more familiar with the practices and the sensations they generate, you will develop the ability to read your own energy system, get feedback, and correct it if it is imbalanced.

GENERAL GUIDELINES

Do:
- *Set time aside so that you will not be interrupted.*
- *Practise in a natural setting whenever you can. You can benefit from the energy of nature.*
- *Find somewhere beautiful and inspiring. At the very least, try to be exposed to sunlight.*
- *Practise with an empty bladder and bowel.*
- *Practise early in the morning, just after waking up.*
- *Practise at night, just before going to sleep.*
- *Practise with your best attention. Approach it with the same sense of respect and reverence as if you were in a church, temple or sacred place (you are!).*

Don't:
- *Practise immediately after a big meal.*
- *Practise if you are exhausted — get some rest first.*
- *Overdo it if you are sick or unwell. Take it easily, gently and lightly, until your strength gradually returns and you feel able to resume normal practice.*

WHAT NEXT?

You will experience your own Qi by doing the exercises on the following pages. Practise them regularly and in a manner which suits you. Select one or two that you find particularly helpful and develop a daily Qi Gong practice; you will quickly find that this develops your Qi and how you experience it.

To continue further, it is advisable to find a qualified teacher and undergo personal training; ask friends for recommendations if you can. A Qi Gong teacher will be known by the quality and volume of their energy, the results that they achieve and their ability to transmit their knowledge to students (see page 157 for recommended teachers). You will be given personalized instructions and experience the teacher's energy — and you will get feedback, which is important for your learning process.

Develop your Qi and you will establish a solid foundation for your health and well-being. You will be healthier and feel better. You will live longer and be happier. Your life will be more successful and you will be of greater value to yourself, your family and friends, and others. Qi Gong is a process of personal and social evolution. Practise Qi Gong, learn how to generate, use and control your energy, and you will cultivate your life.

QUIESCENT QI GONG
Gathering energy at your navel

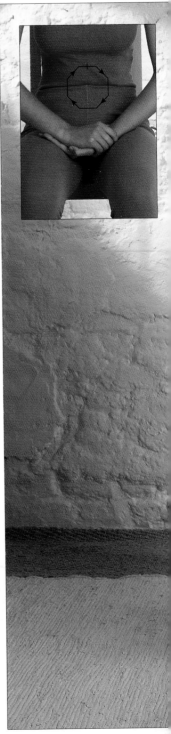

BECOMING AWARE

OF YOUR

INTERNAL ENERGY

This practice quietens your mind and allows you to concentrate and focus your energy. You can do it on its own as a meditation practice, or as a preparation or ending for other Qi Gong practices. It will increase your Qi and allow you to become aware of your internal energy. It will keep you 'centred' by bringing energy to your physical centre. It is a foundation practice common to many forms of Qi Gong, and is one version of Quiescent Qi Gong, becoming quiet. Your navel is the safest place for your energy; it is 'Home Base'.

Sit on the edge of a chair in an upright position, with your knees shoulder-width apart and parallel, and your feet flat on the floor (you can lie down if you prefer). Place your left hand in your lap facing upwards, and your right hand on top of it facing downwards, with the centre of your palms opposite each other. Let your clasped hands rest gently in your lap. This seals in your Qi.

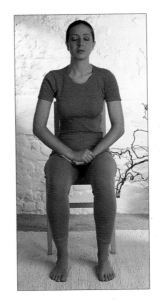

1 PREPARATION
Close your eyes, quieten your mind and breathe deeply. Allow your mind to settle and calm itself. Visualize a cloudless blue sky. Breathe deeply; count your breathing in and out. Allow it to slow down. Place your attention into your navel and begin to draw external energy into it. Continue until it feels warm or until you feel some other sensation there.

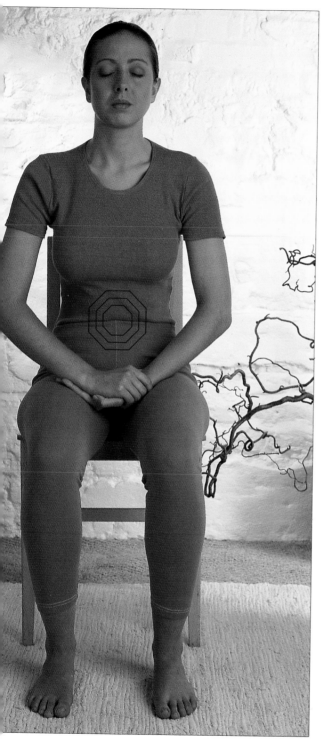

2 FORMING THE BA GUA

You are now going to visualize a Ba Gua – three concentric octagons – around your navel. In this exercise, the outer octagon of the Ba Gua is 7–8 cm (3 in) wide; inside that is a 5 cm (2 in) wide octagon; and finally, there is a 2–3 cm (1 in) wide octagon in the centre. The important point with visualizations is to 'feel' their presence. Do not worry if you do not 'see' clearly. With practice, the mind becomes more stable and can hold visualizations more clearly.

Imagine you are holding a soft, thick felt-tip pen. To begin, start at a level 4 cm (1 ¹/₂ in) above the middle of your navel. Always 'draw' to the left and continue round the octagon in a clockwise direction (see inset left). Repeat this pattern starting 2–3 cm (1 in), and finally 1 cm (¹/₂ in), from your navel.

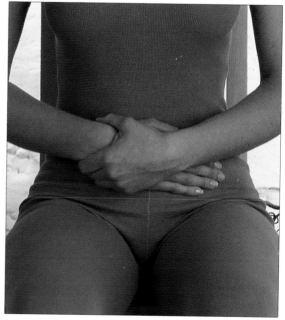

3 SEALING

To seal it, place the centre of one palm over your navel with the centre of the other palm on top of it – left hand first for men, right hand first for women. Concentrate on this area and breathe into it. By developing control over your Ba Gua you gain control over your entire energy and can bring it into your physical centre: your navel. You will feel calm, grounded, alert and relaxed.

CLEANSING
The Fusion of the Five Elements

PURIFY NEGATIVE ENERGY

TO CULTIVATE

'GOODNESS'

The Fusion of the Five Elements is part of what is known as 'Inner Alchemy', the aspect of Qi Gong involved with 'internal transformation'. This practice takes the negative energy of the five major emotions of fear, anxiety, anger, grief and worry out of each of the five organs and purifies them, providing the basis for cultivation of the virtues of each respective organ; together these total 'Goodness'.

The Fusion of the Five Elements is a practical way to cultivate your Goodness. It is like a complete, comprehensive system of psychotherapy, which you do by yourself. A simplified version of this profound practice is given here.

Sit in a comfortable and relaxed position, close your eyes and allow your mind to settle. Place your attention at your navel, and draw a Ba Gua as described previously. Concentrate your energy there. You are now ready to purify and fuse the five elements in your navel; focus on the organs in the order indicated *(see right)*.

After this, return to each cleansed organ, focus your attention there and hold it. Allow the positive virtue to arise and feed it into the next organ, following the Shen (organ generation) cycle: kindness (Kidneys), gentleness (Liver), honour and respect (Heart), fairness (Spleen), righteousness (Lungs). This is the foundation of all higher practices.

1 THE KIDNEYS: PURIFYING FEAR
- *Place your attention into your Kidneys.*
- *The negative emotions are fear, self-consciousness, paranoia.*
- *Feel the quality of the Qi in your Kidneys. Feel the cold-black-fear energy in the Kidneys being drawn out and released. Bring this fear energy from the Kidneys into the Ba Gua at your navel and hold it there.*

2 THE HEART: PURIFYING ANXIETY
- *Place your attention into your Heart (which includes the Pericardium).*
- *The negative emotions are anxiety, hastiness, impatience.*
- *Using your mind, draw the hot-red-anxiety energy out of your Heart into the Ba Gua at your navel and hold it there.*

3 CLEANSE FEAR AND ANXIETY IN THE BA GUA
Now, activate your Ba Gua as if it is an energy vortex. Feel the fear and anxiety being mixed together and broken down into their purified components, just as a poison can be broken down into harmless molecules. Pay attention to how your purified energy now feels.

4 THE LIVER: PURIFYING ANGER
- *Place your attention into your Liver.*
- *The negative emotions are anger, frustration, resentment.*
- *Feel the warm-green-anger energy in the Liver being drawn out and released. Bring this anger energy from the Liver into the Ba Gua at your navel and hold it there.*

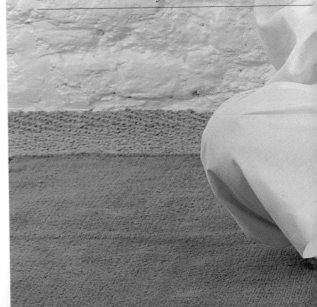

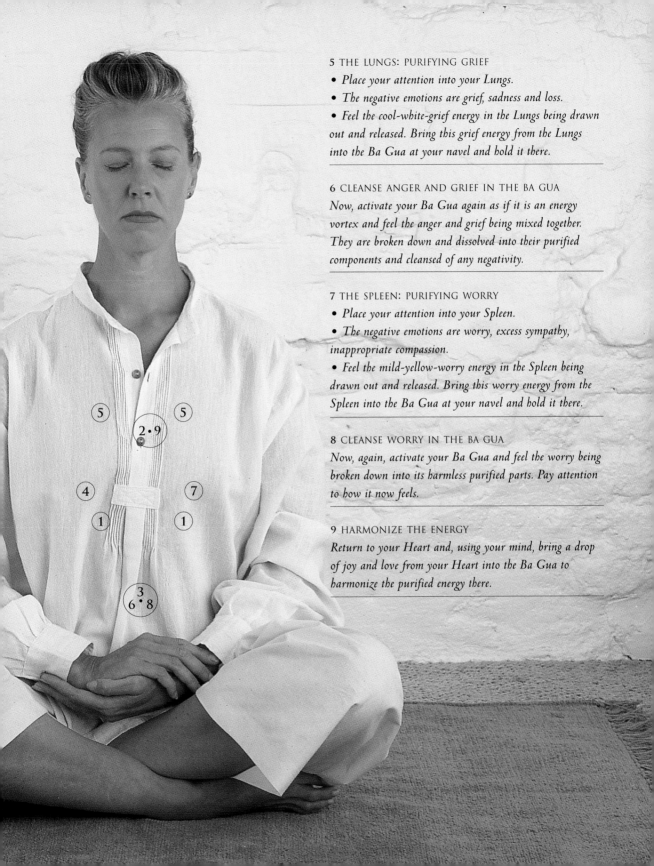

5 THE LUNGS: PURIFYING GRIEF

- *Place your attention into your Lungs.*
- *The negative emotions are grief, sadness and loss.*
- *Feel the cool-white-grief energy in the Lungs being drawn out and released. Bring this grief energy from the Lungs into the Ba Gua at your navel and hold it there.*

6 CLEANSE ANGER AND GRIEF IN THE BA GUA

Now, activate your Ba Gua again as if it is an energy vortex and feel the anger and grief being mixed together. They are broken down and dissolved into their purified components and cleansed of any negativity.

7 THE SPLEEN: PURIFYING WORRY

- *Place your attention into your Spleen.*
- *The negative emotions are worry, excess sympathy, inappropriate compassion.*
- *Feel the mild-yellow-worry energy in the Spleen being drawn out and released. Bring this worry energy from the Spleen into the Ba Gua at your navel and hold it there.*

8 CLEANSE WORRY IN THE BA GUA

Now, again, activate your Ba Gua and feel the worry being broken down into its harmless purified parts. Pay attention to how it now feels.

9 HARMONIZE THE ENERGY

Return to your Heart and, using your mind, bring a drop of joy and love from your Heart into the Ba Gua to harmonize the purified energy there.

INCREASING AND ACCUMULATING
The Golden Stone Ball

INCREASE YOUR ENERGY

WHENEVER YOU

NEED A BOOST

This practice uses the energy between your palms to strengthen your Lower Tan Tien, one of the primary energy centres in the body and the home of your Jing. It increases the energy in your whole system, and is good to do when you are feeling tired or depleted, or to give you a boost of energy when needed.

You can repeat this sequence (steps 3–7) three, seven, twenty-one or more times (these numbers are traditionally considered to be auspicious, and so add a certain power to the practice; however, you can do it as many times as you feel comfortable with). Concentrate your attention in the Lower Tan Tien. Build your Jing. Repeat the same sequence, an equal number of times, in the opposite direction.

To prepare for this practice, stand in a relaxed manner, with your feet shoulder-width apart and facing forward, and your arms hanging softly and loosely by your sides. Allow your mind to settle.

1 *Hold your hands in front of you. The tips of your thumbs should touch each other at the top and rest lightly in the navel, with the tips of your index fingers touching below. The point that lies on the centre line of your abdomen in the middle of the space between your fingers and thumbs is the Lower Tan Tien energy field.*

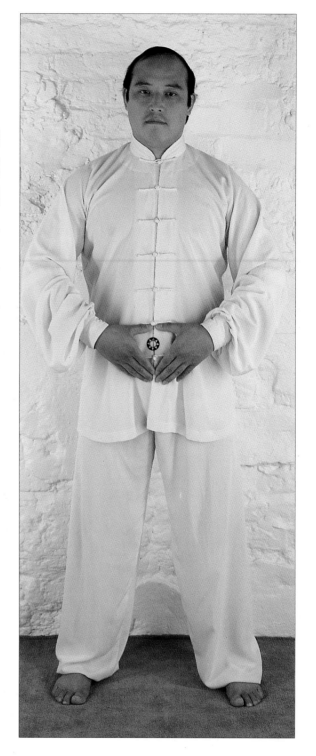

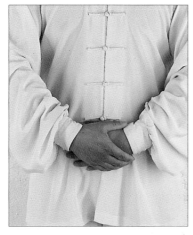

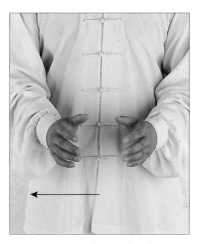

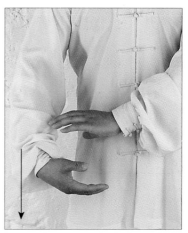

2 Having located the Lower Tan Tien, now hold your hands over it, with both your palms facing inwards (the left hand should be underneath for men, the right hand underneath for women). Feel energy and warmth accumulate in this energy centre.

3 Turn your palms so that they are facing each other about 10–15 cm (4–6 in) apart, as if you were holding a 'Golden Ball'. Feel warmth and Qi accumulate between your palms. Raise them to the level of your navel and draw both hands to the right.

4 Now, turn the ball so that your right palm is below, facing upwards, and your left palm is above, facing downwards. Then, lower the ball in a straight line, down to the level where your index fingers first reached, below the Tan Tien.

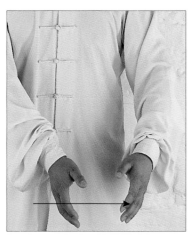

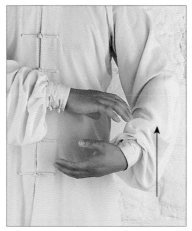

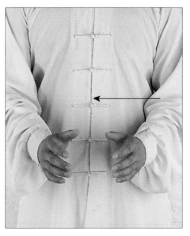

5 Once you have lowered the ball, turn your hands so that your palms are facing each other again. Now bring them across from the right to the left; this is the bottom of the 'square' that you are currently in the process of forming around your Lower Tan Tien.

6 Now turn your palms so that your right palm is on top, facing downwards, and your left palm is underneath, facing upwards. They should still be the same distance apart. Slowly draw them up, vertically, until they are level with your navel.

7 Turn your palms to face each other, then bring them across to the right to complete a square around the lower energy field. Repeat this sequence the same number of times in both directions. To close, place both hands over the Tan Tien, as in step 2; concentrate your energy there.

SELF-MASSAGE
Massaging along your meridians

STIMULATE YOUR ENERGY

TO MAINTAIN SMOOTH

CIRCULATION

Self-massage along the meridians (channels) stimulates your energy circulation, removes obstructions to the flow of Qi and breaks up congestion and blockages. It activates the whole circulation of your channels and keeps your energy flowing smoothly and evenly.

You can do this practice sitting or standing. Allow your mind to settle; your eyes can be open or closed. Concentrate your Qi into your palms. Gently, slowly and firmly run your palms over your meridian pathways in the sequence shown (without making contact with your body) – first one side and then the other. Imagine you are breathing out through your palms, 'dragging' the Qi along the channels.

VARIATIONS

Be creative with this practice; do it:
• *At different speeds and intensities: fast, slow, light, heavy.*
• *Down the inside of both arms, then up the outside; down the outside of both legs, then up the inside.*
• *Using both hands together on your torso, back and legs.*
• *With just your mind.*
• *In co-ordination with your breathing.*
• *Once, or for as long as you like.*
• *Like a slow-motion dance.*
• *To someone else.*

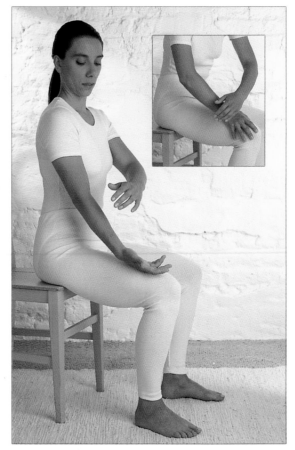

1 *To begin, run your palm from your torso down the inside of your arm to your hand (see above). This stimulates the Heart, Pericardium and Lung channels.*

2 *From the ends of your fingers up the outside of your arm to your head (see inset above). Continue over the top of your head, as shown in the inset above right. This activates the Small Intestine, Triple Burner and Large Intestine channels.*

3 *From the head, back across the body and down the outside and back of your leg to your foot (see right). This moves the Urinary Bladder, Gall Bladder and Stomach channels. Bring your palm right down to the ends of your toes and across to the inner side of your foot. (Note: the next part of the sequence is shown on the opposite leg for maximum clarity; you should continue on the inside of the same leg.)*

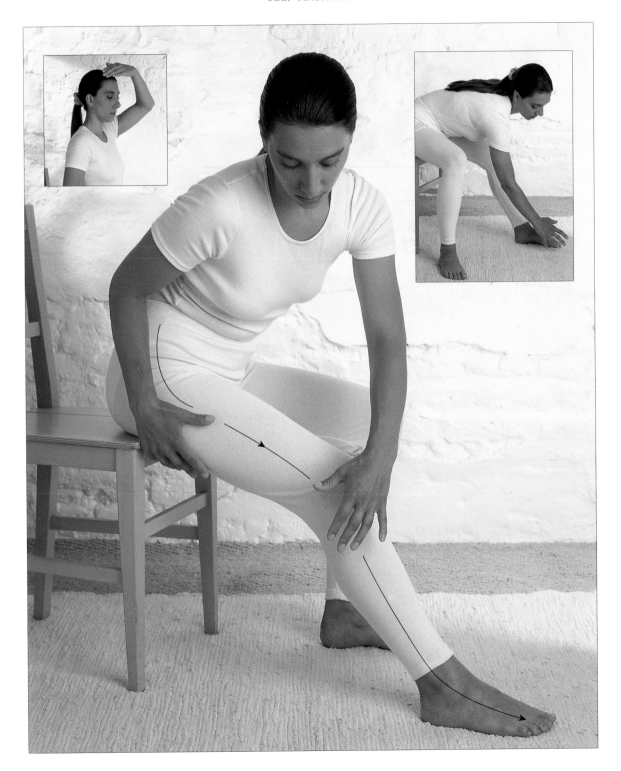

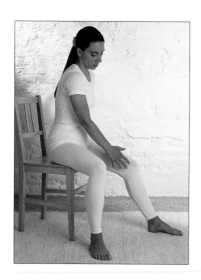

4 From the ends of the toes, up the inside of the leg to the torso. This energizes the Kidney, Liver and Spleen channels (see left).

5 The sequence is complete when you return your palm to your torso (see right). You can repeat the sequence as many times as you like before completion, but make sure you do it the same number of times on both sides of the body.

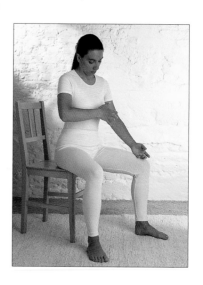

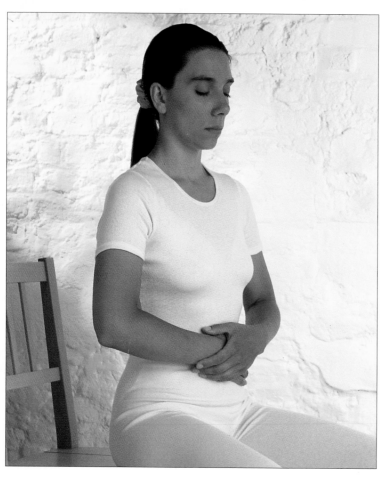

6 COMPLETION
Once you have performed this sequence as many times as you wish, bring both hands and the Palace of Labour points in the palms (point P8 – see page 66) over your Ba Gua at the navel (remember: left hand first for men, right hand first for women). Concentrate your mind there to bring you back to your centre. Pay attention to how you feel, and remember this. You have now used the energy in your palms to move the energy in your channels, controlled and directed by your mind.

EXTERNAL QI GONG
The Three Tan Tien

ENERGIZE, RECHARGE AND

BALANCE YOURSELF

TO FACE THE DAY

This exercise energizes you and makes you ready to face whatever the day holds in store. It brings clean, fresh external energy into you, and builds up and balances your three major energy centres – Jing, Qi and Shen (Essence, Energy and Spirit). It also cleans out stale, negative energy from your system. It is good to do just after getting up or after a shower, but you can also do it any time simply to recharge and balance yourself.

Follow the instructions carefully. When you have learnt the practice and feel comfortable with it, do it according to how you feel and what you need at the time.

To prepare, stand in a relaxed manner with your knees slightly bent and your shoulders loose. Allow your hands to hang by your sides. Close your eyes and allow your mind to settle. Pay attention to how you feel. Relax. Breathe slowly and deeply into your lower abdomen.

When you have completed steps 1–7, bring your palms back to cover your navel, one over the other, as shown in step 1. This point is CV8 *(see page 66)*. Focus your attention here, and slowly breathe in and out, feeling the area under your palms gently expand and contract as you do so. Concentrate your energy there and focus on the sensations generated. When you feel ready, open your eyes very slowly and return to the outside. You can now start the day recharged and refreshed.

1 GATHERING YOUR ENERGY AT YOUR NAVEL

Place your hands directly over your navel, one hand on top of the other, so that the energy point located in the centre of your palms is aligned with your navel. For men the left hand should be on the bottom, touching the navel, with the right hand on top of it, and the other way round for women.

Focus on this point in the centre of your palms and breathe slowly in and out. Draw external energy through this point into your navel; feel it grow warmer, brighter, fuller, lighter.

77

2 GATHERING EXTERNAL QI FROM HEAVEN

Slowly draw your arms up, out to the sides, then turn your palms face up. As you breathe in, use your mind to draw external energy into them from sky, sun, moon, stars and heaven.

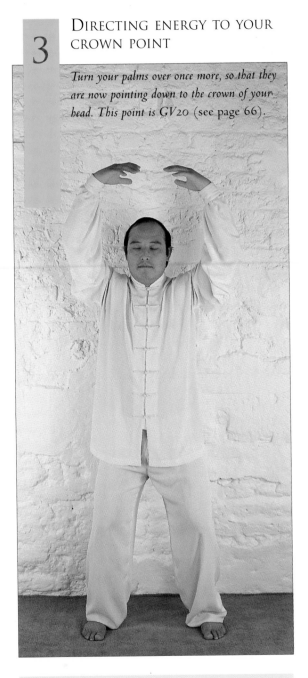

As you breathe out, disconnect your mind to keep this energy in your palms. Draw in more energy as you breathe in. Repeat for three breaths, or until your palms are full of energy.

3 DIRECTING ENERGY TO YOUR CROWN POINT

Turn your palms over once more, so that they are now pointing down to the crown of your head. This point is GV20 (see page 66).

Direct the energy from your palms here as you breathe out. Let your energy radiate to your crown; place your attention there and feel the energy increase. Repeat for three breaths.

4 BRINGING YOUR ENERGY TO THE UPPER TAN TIEN

Slowly bring your arms and hands down in front of you, palms facing you, fingertips 8–10 cm (3–4 in) apart, until the point in the centre of each palm is level with, and facing, the point on the mid-line between your eyebrows (Yintang — see page 66). This is the Upper Tan Tien, the centre of Shen.

5 BRINGING YOUR ENERGY TO THE MIDDLE TAN TIEN

Slowly bring your arms and hands down in front of you, palms facing towards you, until the point in the centre of your palms is level with, and facing, the centre of your chest. This point is CV17 (see page 66), the Middle Tan Tien. It is the home of your Qi.

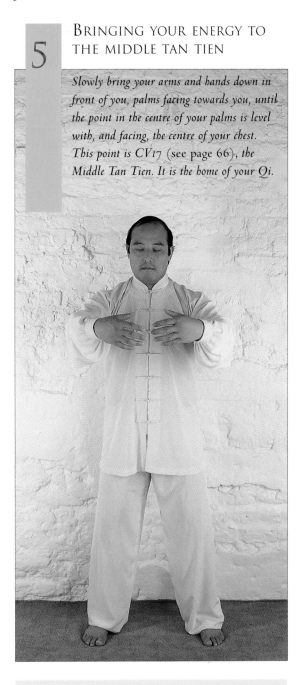

As you slowly breathe out, direct your energy to this point; it activates your brain and mind. Be aware of it and feel the energy increase there. Repeat for three breaths.

This point activates, stimulates and develops the Heart, the thymus gland and the immune system. As you breathe out, direct your energy here. Repeat for three breaths.

6 BRINGING YOUR ENERGY TO THE LOWER TAN TIEN

Again, slowly bring your arms and hands down in front of you, palms facing towards you, until they are opposite the point 5–7 cm (2–3 in) below your navel. This is CV6 (see page 66).

7 SENDING YOUR ENERGY OUT THROUGH YOUR FEET

Slowly continue down with your palms and hands, directing the Qi from the centre of your palms down through your lower torso. Allow your arms to hang gently by your sides. With your mind, continue down through your legs and then out through the point at the soles of your feet (K1 – see page 66).

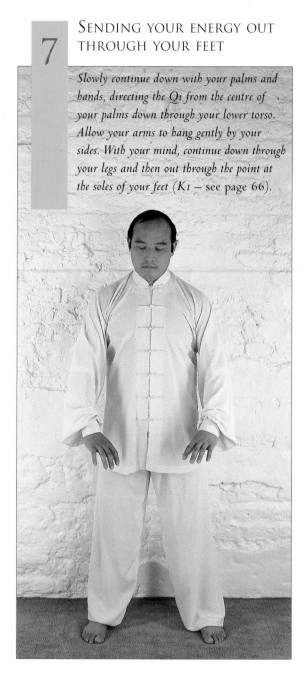

This area, the Lower Tan Tien, is the home and foundation of your Jing. As you slowly breathe out, direct your energy to this point. Repeat this for three breaths.

Continue to direct your Qi down to one metre (3 feet) below you. This helps to clean out stale or negative energy from your system, and sends it outside your personal energy field.

INTERNAL QI GONG
The Microcosmic Orbit

ACTIVATE YOUR INTERNAL

ENERGY CENTRES AND

INTEGRATE YOUR SYSTEM

The circuit which runs up and down the front and back centre-line of the body is known as the Microcosmic Orbit. It is one of the primary circuits in Qi Gong training and is common to all forms, styles and traditions of Qi Gong because it co-ordinates and integrates all of the other energy channels in the body. It is of special significance as it utilizes the Conception Vessel and Governor Vessel channels; these are two of the Eight Extra Channels *(see page 24)*. The energy points that are used relate to, and activate, the deeper-level internal centres known as the 'Cauldrons' (chakras).

This practice integrates the whole system and is a basic requirement for higher levels of Inner Alchemy training. At first, practise lightly and gently, then slowly increase duration and intensity as you develop. Hold your attention at each of the specified points for the same amount of time and the same number of breaths.

Later, as you become more experienced and your sensitivity heightens, you will develop the ability to 'read' how your energy is at any given point, and to hold it there for greater or shorter periods of time, as needed. With that experience, you can repeat this sequence for varying amounts of time or hold your attention for differing numbers of breaths at each point.

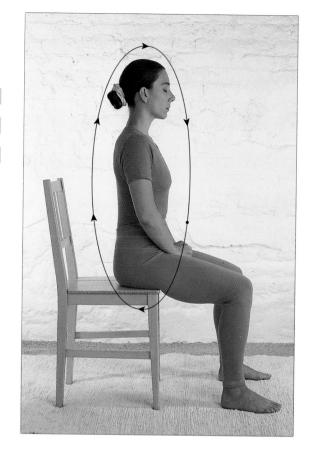

1 PREPARATION
Sit on the edge of a chair. Relax your neck and shoulders. Your back should be straight so that Qi and Blood may circulate without obstruction. If you have a back problem, sit whichever way is most comfortable. Make sure that your feet are flat on the ground facing forward, and are shoulder-width apart. Clasp your palms in front of you — left facing up and right facing down on top of left. Close your eyes and put your attention inside yourself. Form a Ba Gua around your navel (see pages 68–69), and hold your mind there until you begin to experience warmth and energy. You are about to focus your attention on points in your body which make up a complete circuit — the Microcosmic Orbit — as shown above on the picture above.

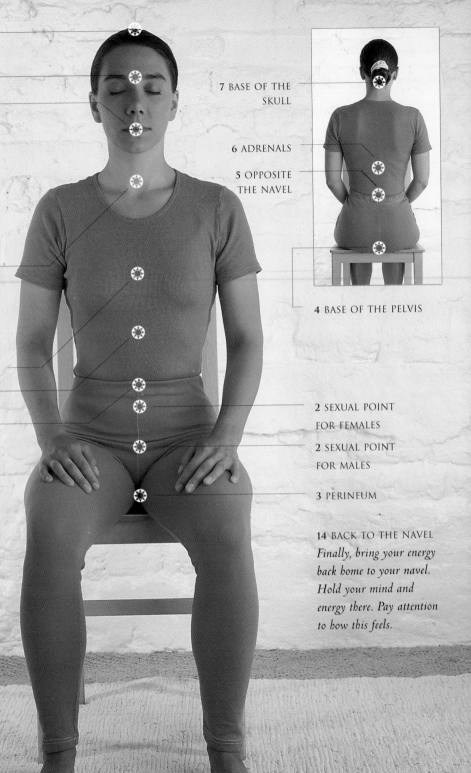

8 CROWN OF THE HEAD

9 BROW

10 ROOF OF THE MOUTH
Now, connect the tip of your tongue to the roof of your mouth behind the upper teeth. You may feel a tingling sensation. This connects the Governor Vessel to the Conception Vessel.

11 THROAT
Bring your attention down through your tongue and throat to the point just below your Adam's Apple.

12 CENTRE OF THE CHEST

13 SOLAR PLEXUS

1 NAVEL
Place your attention into your navel. Imagine that you are drawing Qi in and out through your navel until you begin to feel an energy sensation there: this may feel warm, full or tingling, or perhaps a different sensation. This procedure has opened up your energy at your navel and turned it on.

7 BASE OF THE SKULL

6 ADRENALS

5 OPPOSITE THE NAVEL

4 BASE OF THE PELVIS

2 SEXUAL POINT FOR FEMALES

2 SEXUAL POINT FOR MALES

3 PERINEUM

14 BACK TO THE NAVEL
Finally, bring your energy back home to your navel. Hold your mind and energy there. Pay attention to how this feels.

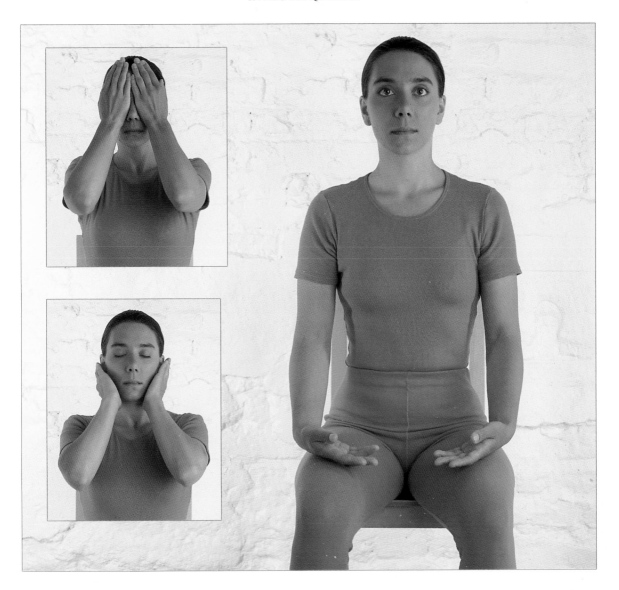

2 FOCUSING YOUR ATTENTION

You are now going to bring your attention to different points along the circuit in turn (follow the order given — see left). When you do so, breathe in and out three or more times, using the same number of breaths at each point. Hold your mind, your attention and your concentration at the point, and this will focus your energy there (concentrate in the general area). Keep your hands clasped in your lap throughout (they are shown here resting on the thighs so the points can be seen).

3 SEALING YOUR ENERGY

To end, seal your energy back into your navel (see step 6 on page 76). Then, rub your palms together and place them over your eyes (see top inset). Feel their warmth calm and refresh your eyes. Now wash your face with the energy in your palms (see bottom inset). Finally, rest your hands on your thighs, slowly open your eyes and return to awareness of your surroundings. Your energy is now moving as it should: feel it, work with it, develop it, cultivate it — and enjoy it.

CHAPTER FIVE

CHINESE MASSAGE

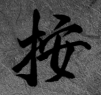

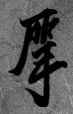

- *The power of Chinese massage*
- *Development of domestic and clinical techniques*
- *The benefits of An Mo massage*
- *An Mo massage routine to practise at home*
- *Children's Chinese massage*

Chinese massage therapy is very different to the type of massage practised in the West. At a professional level, it is used to treat specific imbalances of Qi and Blood diagnosed by the practitioner. At a more everyday level, the techniques are used to strengthen Qi and Blood and to help them flow harmoniously around the body. Most people in China use massage regularly to maintain health and to treat minor symptoms. The methods given here can be easily applied to your friends and relatives so that they too can experience their benefits.

CHINESE MASSAGE IN ACTION

The following story demonstrates just how powerful Chinese massage can be. A woman travelling on a train in China suddenly felt intense pain under her ribs. It radiated around her flanks to the middle of her back and was so severe that she could not bring herself to move. The guard was summoned and he, in turn, located a doctor of Western medicine at the other end of the train. The doctor diagnosed acute pain from gallstones, but had no drugs with him to alleviate the woman's suffering, nor any equipment with which to operate. In any case, the train was hardly the most sterile environment.

The train sped onwards, and a doctor of Chinese acupuncture then came on the scene. She made a diagnosis of gallstones due to DampHeat in the Liver and Gall Bladder. She would have inserted needles into various points on the lower ribs and on the legs, but unfortunately she had no needles or any other equipment with her.

A doctor of Chinese massage therapy then heard about the case. He made the same diagnosis as the acupuncturist and decided he

must use certain techniques with his thumb on selected energy points. Fortunately, he had both his thumbs with him and set to work immediately. He applied vigorous 'One-finger-meditation' technique to a Gall Bladder point below the knee for a good forty-five minutes with his right thumb, while alternating his other thumb between points on the left and right sides at the woman's twelfth rib.

When the train reached its destination the woman was virtually pain-free and was able to walk to a nearby hospital of Chinese medicine for further examination and treatment.

This story illustrates three points:

• Chinese massage therapy can be given at any time and in any place without the need for any equipment at all.

• It is not in any way inferior to acupuncture in treating even internal diseases.

• If other points and techniques had been used or only a general massage given, the treatment would have been next to useless in the circumstances. Chinese massage therapy is accurate if done correctly, according to a proper Chinese diagnosis.

HISTORY

The earliest surviving reference to massage in China is in the 'Yellow Emperor's Inner Classic' (*Huangdi Neijing*). This text mentions twelve different massage techniques and their clinical applications. However, earlier texts on massage did exist, as proved by reference to them in later works. Massage in these earlier times was usually referred to as An Mo, literally 'pressing and rubbing', after two common massage techniques.

From as early as the second century AD, Chinese herbal prescriptions in ointment form were used for specific An Mo treatments. This involved the application of herbal ointments, which had been tailored to the task according to the diagnosis, to areas of the body or to specific points for both internal and superficial diseases.

PERIODS OF FLOURISHING

During the Tang dynasty (AD 618–906), an An Mo section was set up within the Imperial Medical offices. At this time, An Mo became the primary treatment for children's diseases, a role it still retains today. During this period Japan officially adopted Chinese medicine, including massage therapy, which became known there as *An Ma*.

Amidst military activities in the Song and Yuan periods (AD 960–1368), An Mo massage techniques began to specialize in the treatment of war injuries. The Chinese massage therapy method of bone setting, which allows bones some movement as they heal in position, eliminates many of the post-treatment complications that occur with other methods.

The next great flourishing was in the Ming period (AD 1368–1644), when clinical massage therapy became known as *Tui Na*, literally 'pushing and grabbing', after two of its techniques. From this time onwards, An Mo has referred only to domestic, non-clinical massage.

AN MO AND TUI NA TODAY

Nowadays, An Mo refers exclusively to massage that everyone can do, whether to family at home or to friends at work. It is done for general relaxation, to release the tensions of modern life and to help improve well-being and immunity to disease, thereby giving illness less of a chance to develop. An Mo can also be beneficial in treating many common complaints. In addition, children respond well to massage and thoroughly enjoy it; in China, they begin to receive it from an early age.

Tui Na, on the other hand, refers exclusively to professional, clinical massage therapy as practised by Chinese doctors, either in hospitals of Chinese medicine or in private practices and clinics. Some techniques of Tui Na are extremely difficult and take years to master. Additionally, Tui Na is always done according to a formal Chinese medical diagnosis, and so demands a thorough knowledge of Chinese medicine theory; without this, it simply would not be Tui Na.

THE BENEFITS OF AN MO

The emphasis of An Mo is on helping yourself *before* you become ill or in the early stages of illness, rather than after you have actually developed chronic symptoms. An Mo enhances your psychological state and your immune system by encouraging 'wholesome' responses in your mind and body; touch on the surface of the body can reach the deepest levels of the mind – far deeper than words. Wherever the flow of Qi and Blood is obstructed you will experience pain or discomfort and your system as a whole will malfunction. Massage, more than any other therapy, impacts directly on to the channels producing a healthy flow of Qi and Blood throughout the body. When your channels are regularly cleared and your vital organs bathed in nourishment, you will experience much less discomfort and generally feel healthy and energetic.

The judgemental part of our mind (*see page 49 for further discussion*) constantly responds to sensations with attachment or aversion, liking some and hating others. Whenever this aspect of the mind is agitated (which is virtually all the time, although you may not be aware of it) there will be some kind of sensation on the surface of the body. Likewise, whenever there is a sensation on the surface of the body, the judgemental mind will react by either liking it or hating it. This is what stress really is: your own reaction against the world, rather than the effect of the world itself upon you. This is the reason why meditation is such a highly beneficial practice, because it fundamentally changes our reactions to sensations, whether they come from the external world or from inside ourselves.

By using touch to create sensations on the surface of the body, An Mo encourages emotional states to come up to the surface and disperse rather than stay fermenting and multiplying in the inner depths of the body.

The use of touch given in a loving and compassionate way can generate similar responses in our body and mind.

Kindness and Compassion

The person who gives An Mo massage is giving not only skill but also Qi. Such Qi is received as a 'gift' from the universe, from the food we eat and the air we breathe. Therefore, when someone near you is ill, in discomfort or needs support, it is right that you should share this gift with them. This is the tradition of Chinese medicine which is closely related to spiritual practices of compassion and the desire to relieve suffering. Massage is the most obstacle-free physical way to give your Qi to others, to pour the vibrations generated within you into another person's body.

The quality of Qi that you give is more important than Qi itself. Compassion and loving kindness are the root of healthy Qi. It is helpful to cultivate caring feelings without expecting anything in return when you give An Mo to others. When you give Qi with compassion it has a deeply beneficial physical and psychological influence on the person receiving it and also, just as importantly, on yourself.

One of the effects of An Mo is that the people you give it to feel more well-disposed both towards you and towards the world in general. By developing your own faculty of compassion, you also develop more kindness towards others. There is another phenomenon, too: the giver of An Mo receives compassionate vibrations from the recipient during the massage itself. With such giving and taking being the basis of family relationships and friendship, the only result can be more harmony in life.

AN MO FOR FAMILY AND FRIENDS

What follows is a routine you can do at home in order to give massage to your family and friends. This routine is good for general relaxation and well-being, and for improving immunity to disease. The length of time that the whole routine takes can vary — it can last for as long as the giver and the recipient feel comfortable — but it will generally take from twenty minutes up to an hour *(see also 'Massage Time' below)*. It has been arranged in order of sequence, but each stage represents a different yet common technique of An Mo massage. Each technique has a different function, and once you have become familiar with them you will be able to make your own variations according to your needs. You will find that some techniques appear twice in the sequence: this is because they have beneficial effects at more than one stage in the routine.

Many of the techniques need to be given through loose cotton clothing or through a soft cotton cloth placed over the area to be treated; this is because they would otherwise be fairly rough on the surface of the skin. The use of cotton material is optional for those techniques shown being applied directly on the skin (with the exception of those which use balm or talcum powder — *see information on massage media opposite*); they have been shown here without the use of a cloth for maximum clarity.

MASSAGE TIME

There is no statutory duration for most of the techniques; indeed, to give rigid time schedules would spoil the interaction of awareness between giver and recipient. In any instance, the length of time for which you do each technique should be natural and intuitive — most people are surprised by just how easily this intuition comes. Of course, your intuition will become more finely tuned as you become more experienced.

CAUTIONS

When giving An Mo make sure that you never force anything. Always stay with what you are comfortable with and feel clear about. As you develop your experience, you will automatically increase your range of capability without even trying. In fact, it is this very aspect of *not* trying that will make your An Mo successful. Just as meditation and Qi Gong are states of 'being' rather than 'doing', if you can develop a similar attitude whilst performing An Mo it will be more effective. In such a state, the Qi and Blood flow more harmoniously and this is mirrored in the person receiving An Mo massage.

Before you begin your massage, make sure you are familiar with the information given below on when to seek professional help.

SEEKING PROFESSIONAL HELP

Please bear in mind that An Mo is a preventative treatment rather than a cure. If you are in any doubt about the condition of a person to whom you are going to give An Mo, it is best to consult a practitioner beforehand. He or she will give you guidance on what you can do for your friend or relative at home. For any minor problem that does not respond to An Mo, and for more difficult conditions, it is important to seek the advice of a practitioner fully trained in Tui Na clinical massage and Chinese Medicine *(for more information on Tui Na see page 99)*.

CONTRA-INDICATIONS

There are certain circumstances in which you should not give An Mo and some where you should limit what you do. These are as follows:

• Heart conditions and high blood pressure *Avoid working on the chest, abdomen or upper back so that you do not induce any congestion. The recipient may be more comfortable if his or her trunk is raised with pillows. Restrict your work to the arms, legs and head.*

• Spinal injury *Working on an injured spine is a specialist task. Do not undertake it unless you are fully trained to do so.*

• Cancer *The conventional wisdom is that massage of the cancer itself can accelerate the spread of cancer via blood and lymph. This would be possible if deep massage were given to the sites of the tumours; however, gentle, non-penetrating massage away from the site can harmlessly give incalculable relief from discomfort. Also, laying your palm on the person's belly, either with or without Vibrating technique, can safely bring about considerable relief from the 'whirlpools' in the stomach that often affect cancer sufferers. If you are at all worried about giving massage to someone with cancer, seek professional advice beforehand.*

MASSAGE MEDIA

You do not need a large pharmacy to begin practising ointment massage at home; some common household substances, and others which are easily obtainable, can be used to great effect. A selection is given below.

Toasted sesame oil

This is available in supermarkets, health-food shops and Chinese and Asian emporia. It has a nourishing action on the digestion and a moistening action on the skin. Use it along either side of the spine and also on the upper belly area in cases of Spleen Qi deficiency, especially in children.

Pure talcum powder

This is available from Chinese pharmacies, herbalists and Tui Na doctors. Talcum has the action of drying Dampness and clearing Summer-heat, and is another excellent medium for children. Use it with Pushing technique to either side of the spine on the lower back in cases of diarrhoea due to Dampness, especially in summer.

Vinegar

Use rice vinegar, available cheaply from Chinese emporia, to treat injury (see page 140). Buffing technique will help the vinegar to penetrate under the skin to relax the sinews, activate the Blood and disperse swellings. Ice-packs may momentarily alleviate the pain but will certainly make the area worse shortly afterwards; ice is cold and so obstructs the smooth flow of Qi. Instead, after An Mo has been given, bathe the affected limb in some warmed rice vinegar for about twenty to thirty minutes. If the area is red, add some crushed gardenia fruit to the vinegar; this has a cooling action and thereby relieves inflammation which manifests as heat and redness.

Balm

Some commonly available Chinese balms can be used to continue acting on a point after the massage is finished. Essential Balm is good for this when applied with Kneading technique, and it has a pleasant fragrance. Tiger Balm can also be used in this way, or applied to larger areas. For example, use Burnishing or Buffing technique to areas of musculo-skeletal pain as long as there is no redness on the area.

STROKING

There are two different modes of this technique: strengthening and reducing. The strengthening mode can be used where Spleen Qi is weak, and the reducing mode can be used where there is accumulation of Dampness or stagnation of Qi or food in the abdomen. If there is any evidence of both conditions – Spleen Qi weakness (*see page 35*) with Damp accumulation (*see page 36*) – you should combine both strengthening and reducing modes.

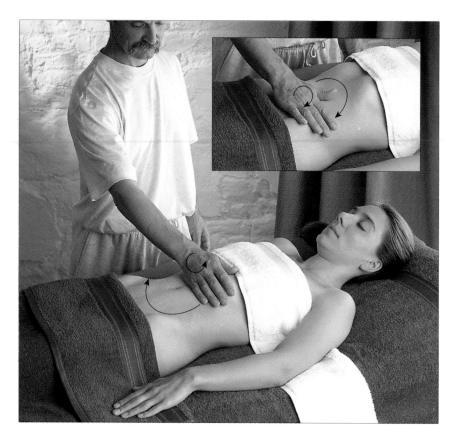

1 Strengthening: *place one of your palms on the upper belly. Begin to rotate your palm anticlockwise in small circles at the rate of two to three rotations per second. This movement should come from your elbow forwards to your hand. At the same time as rotating your hand, let your whole arm move from your shoulder in clockwise direction so that your hand also moves slowly in a wider circle clockwise around the circumference of the belly.*

2 Reducing (see inset): *for this, simply change the direction of the smaller circles to clockwise, so that it is the same direction as the larger circle around the belly.*

BUFFING

This spreads Liver Qi and relieves abdominal distension and ache. The 'buffing' is done by the fleshy pad at the base of the thumb.

3 *Place your hand on the upper belly, just below the ribs. Making a sideways movement from your wrist, let your fingers fly out from side to side creating a fast oscillating movement at the fleshy pad. Let your elbow open out and bend in to direct your hand back and forth across the upper belly.*

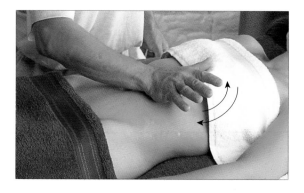

PRESSING

This technique relaxes the sinews and clears obstruction from the channels. The pressing is done using the heels of both palms, which are placed on one of the recipient's thighs, slightly outside of centre, to begin.

4 Lean downwards as you breathe out, transmitting your weight on to the thigh; as you breathe in, release the pressure. Keeping one hand at the top of the thigh, move the other hand down a little, and repeat this procedure down to the knee.

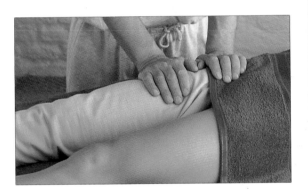

KNEADING

This relaxes the sinews, clears obstruction, invigorates Blood flow, dissolves masses and stops pain. The Chinese way of kneading dough is to use a circular pressing with the hand rather than rotating the dough itself, and this is what is done in this technique.

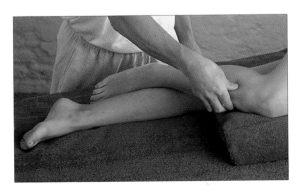

5 As you switch from the thigh to the lower leg, move your non-working hand down to the top of the lower leg. Continue pressing down the leg, and when you have finished slide your static hand down to the foot, keeping it there as you move round to the other side. Then start again on the other thigh with your previously static hand.

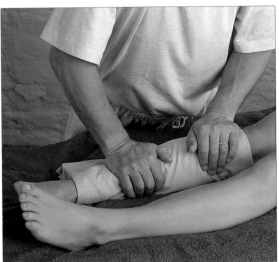

The pressure must be strong so as to break down the gluten vertically, and the circular direction ensures that it is broken down laterally as well as making sure that the entire area is covered. Kneading is done in three main ways: with the thumb, with the middle finger underneath the index finger of the same hand, and with the heel of the palm.

Press down hard to produce the ache known as De Qi, 'obtaining the Qi', which means that you have successfully activated the point and Qi is present. This sensation might be a numbness or tingling, or an 'electric' feeling. The stronger the sensation, the stronger the Qi.

6 Use your thumb to knead GB34 (see page 27). This smooths the flow of Liver Qi and relaxes the tendons (the other two methods of Kneading are featured on page 95).

ROWING

This opens up the channels that pass through the shoulder joints allowing Qi to flow freely between the upper extremities and the rest of the body. When you row a boat, the oar is held at a pivot point while the hand holding the end moves in a rounded motion. Similarly, this technique is given to the arms, with the recipient sitting upright. Repeat steps 7–9 three to four times on one arm, then work on the other arm following the same procedure, but with your hands the other way round.

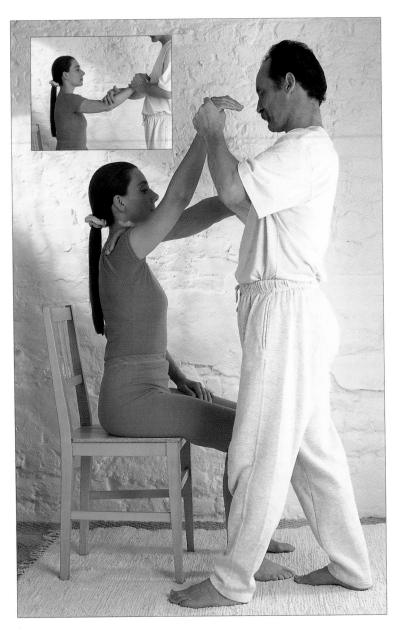

7 Stand facing the recipient and hold their right wrist in your left hand, with your right hand loosely around their forearm. Draw the arm towards you to start (see inset). Step forward so that the arm is raised, and slide your right hand down to the shoulder.

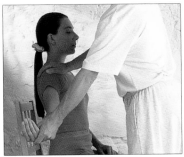

8 Hold the shoulder firm as you step further forward to bring the arm to a point where you feel slight resistance.

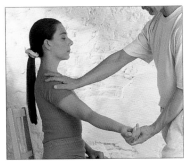

9 Now step backwards, drawing the arm down and back towards you as your right hand slides back down to the forearm again.

GRABBING

This technique has different effects depending on where it is done; Grabbing the limbs simply relaxes the muscles in the area, whereas the effects of Grabbing on specific points will be according to the function of the point concerned. Grabbing technique is done with either three or five fingers, depending on the area being treated – five-finger Grabbing is used for larger areas. Grabbing technique used on the two points mentioned here is particularly helpful.

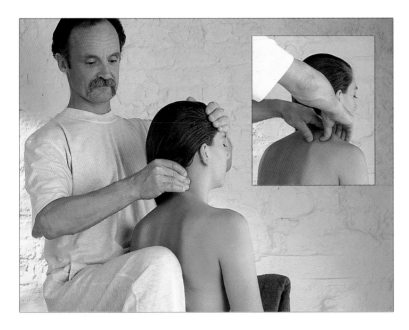

10 *Use your thumb, middle and fourth fingers to grab the muscles at the back of the neck on point GB20 (see page 28); keep your fingers straight or you may hurt the recipient. As soon as the grabbing action has been made, release your grip. Repeat this process until the area being treated feels more freed up to the recipient. Grabbing this area relieves the neck, smooths Liver Qi and brightens the eyes.*

11 *Use all five fingers to grab GB21 (see page 28) to regulate Qi and Blood in the channels (see inset). Again, keep your fingers straight and do not grab too hard.*

RUBDOWN

Done on the flanks, Rubdown smooths the flow of Qi in the chest and lower ribs. It can also be used on the limbs to relax the muscles. The recipient should wear a loose-fitting cotton top for this technique (if he or she is not wearing one already). In Chinese, the word for Rubdown also describes 'rubbing the hands together'; it conveys the mutually opposite motion of the hands, as in this technique.

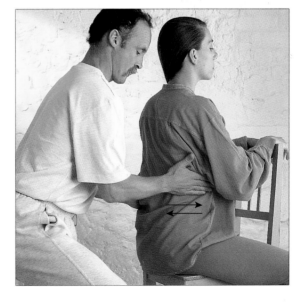

12 *Standing behind your seated recipient, make your hands and fingers tight and straight and place them on the flanks. With a very fast motion back and forth – your hands moving opposite directions – rub the flanks vigorously. Make sure the pressure is neither too hard not too soft.*

BURNISHING

This technique scatters Cold, releases the exterior levels of the body and raises the clear Yang (the good, pure Yang energy). For this technique, the recipient should have their back and upper buttocks completely bare, and you will need some massage medium such as pure talcum powder or balm (*see page* 89). Your palm should be in contact with the person's skin but there should be no pressure; use your right hand if you are right-handed, and your left if you are left-handed. If you press down you will not create much warmth on the body, whereas if you use a light touch you will create great heat with only three or four strokes, which is sufficient.

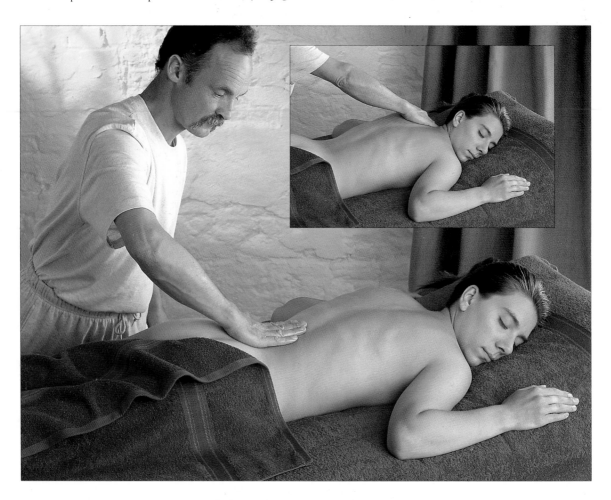

13 *Apply some of the chosen medium to your hand and, to begin with, smear it along the spine and to either side of it. Now, with the palm of your hand lying on the upper buttock, rapidly move your hand along one side of the spine all the way up to point GB21 (see page 28) and back* *again. The momentum should come from your shoulder joint and the movement should be very rapid and follow the contours of the body everywhere along the way. When you have finished doing Burnishing technique on one side of the spine, do it on the other side still using the same hand.*

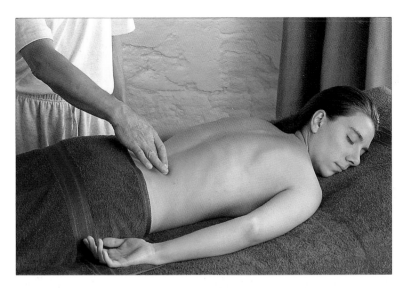

14 KNEADING
You have already used your thumb in this technique on the leg. Now try kneading on point UB23 (see page 28) using your index finger on top of your middle finger of the same hand (see left). This strengthens the Kidney. Remember to apply a strong downward pressure throughout the circular kneading motion.

15 *Now try it with the heel of your palm on the point UB18 (see page 28). This strengthens and regulates the Liver (see below).*

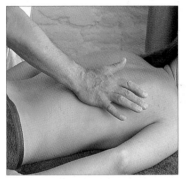

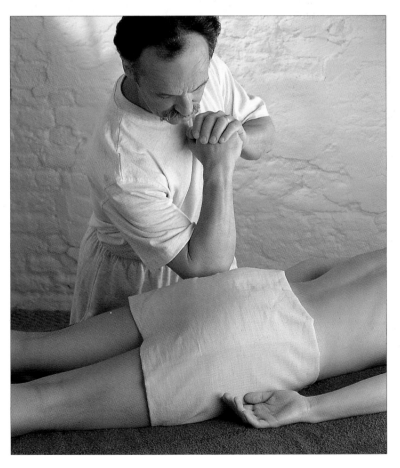

16 SUPPRESSING
This is a heavier version of Pressing which uses the elbow instead of the hands. Place your elbow in the circular depression on the side of the buttock (GB30 – see page 27) and press down. If the depression is not visible, ask the recipient to roll on to their side and bend their upper leg so that you can locate it. Suppressing should bring about a strong sensation of 'obtaining the Qi'; it can also be done on GB30 for blockage at the hip or pain that radiates down the leg.

17 GRABBING
Do Grabbing with
five fingers all along the
backs of the recipient's legs
to release the muscles. Your
grabbing action should be
firm in order to have an
effect. At the same time, be
aware of the recipient's
feelings; the technique should
give no more than a faint,
therapeutic ache.

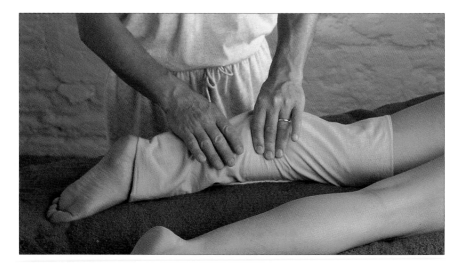

18 PRESSING
Smooth off the legs
by Pressing with the heels of
your palms all along the
backs of the legs. It is
helpful to do Pressing again
at this stage in the routine
to relax the sinews and clear
any obstructions from the
channels. This simple
technique can be widely used
on many parts of the body.
Try to use your body's
weight to give pressure
naturally. This will produce
a much deeper effect than
using your own muscle
power to bear down.

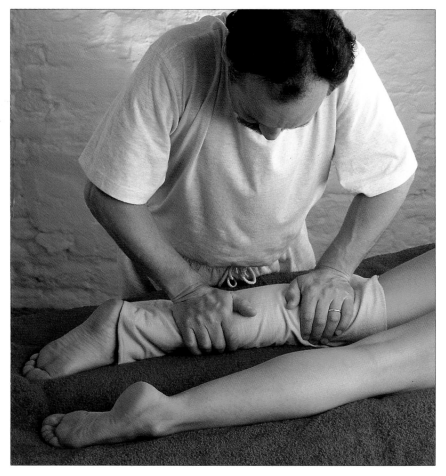

19 BUFFING

This technique used on the face activates the Qi and Blood in the channels. The recipient will need to roll over on to their back again at this point. Place the fleshy pad at the base of your thumb on to the forehead and, with a sideways movement from the wrist, as before, do Buffing technique from one side of the forehead to the other (see right). Then, continue down each cheek before moving back to the centre of the forehead to finish (see below). Although your hand should oscillate quite fast, your touch should be light and easy. Be careful not to let your fingers strike the recipient as you go.

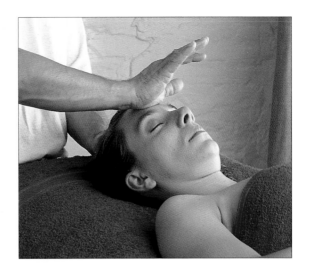

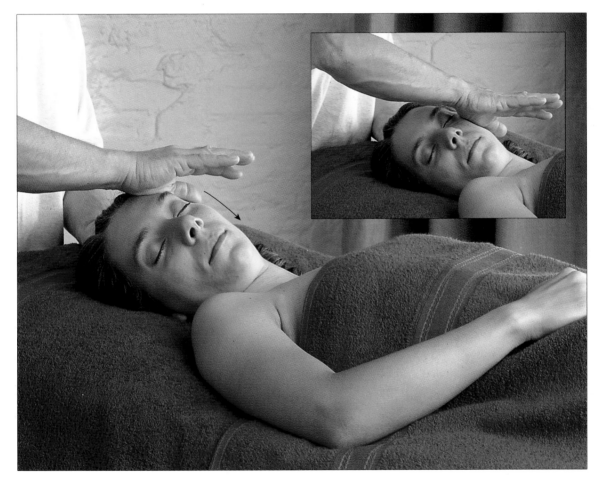

VIBRATING

This technique activates points and regulates Qi in the internal organs. Used on the upper belly, Vibrating alleviates stomach aches and distension; on the lower belly it is very useful for menstrual pains and cramps (it can also be used on the chest to help open stuffy sensations in the upper trunk). Your recipient will experience this technique as a deep, inner vibration.

To create the 'vibrating' sensation, first you need to make your fingers tight, straight and hard but do not press down in the slightest way. Then make your whole arm as tight and hard as you can using every muscle in it to the maximum. Make everything so tight that your arm actually begins to vibrate. The direction of the vibration should be up and down, not side to side, and should only just be visible to the eye and no more.

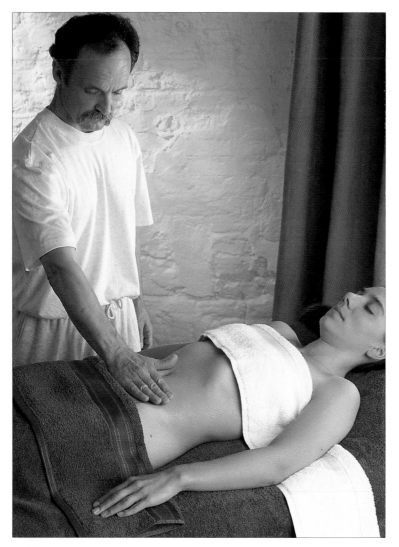

20 Stand or kneel beside the recipient's hip and place your hand on either the lower or upper belly area (see left). Then tighten your arm and fingers, as described above, to create the vibration. The recipient will sense this vibrating deep inside their belly.

21 Now move down towards the feet and place your index finger on top of your middle finger on point Sp6 (see page 27); you can do this on one Sp6 point at a time or, if you feel able, on both Sp6 points together, using both your hands. Again, use Vibrating technique to activate this strengthening, soothing point subtly.

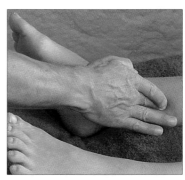

TUI NA: CLINICAL MASSAGE

In any hospital of Chinese Medicine in China there is always a department of Tui Na, and it is always the most popular department. Although it is more expensive than acupuncture, the queue for Tui Na will often start from 5am to be ready at 8am.

As you have seen from the story included at the beginning of this chapter, Tui Na is used to treat specific diseases. The primary medicine for internal complaints is herbal medicine. Nonetheless, although Tui Na is most often used for musculo-skeletal ailments, those who favour it will also use it for many internal diseases as well.

The techniques of Tui Na mentioned in this chapter are only a selection of those available to the professional. There are many more, some of them easy to acquire and a few of them requiring long practise on a rice-bag before practising on the human body. Professional Tui Na doctors possess an unusual combination of seemingly opposing personal traits. While they share with all doctors of Chinese medicine the rigorous, academic discipline of Chinese diagnosis, it is their sheer love of strenuous physical activity that attracts them to Tui Na. The physical strength which they cultivate is counter-balanced with the perfection of an art and the desire to heal.

All muscle and joint problems respond well to Tui Na, as well as internal disorders ranging from period problems to palpitations. Indeed, with its expertise in all kinds of manipulation, the ancient art of Tui Na can be fairly regarded as the father of osteopathy and chiropractic. Although Tui Na cannot address itself to everything, its range goes far beyond that of many other massage therapies in the world, and as such it constitutes a vital method of treatment in the field of Chinese medicine.

CHILDREN'S CHINESE MASSAGE

Tui Na massage is the principal treatment used for infants and young children in Chinese Medicine, as opposed to herbs or acupuncture, when professional help is sought. From a medical viewpoint, children differ from adults for various reasons; for instance, a child's digestive system constantly has to work to maximum capacity to keep the child growing. This means that any slight overloading on the digestive system will cause it to seize up and form a blockage. From this blockage many problems can arise: constipation, diarrhoea, teething pain, waking at night, tantrums, vomiting, stomach pain — the list goes on. Also, the channels are not yet fully formed, which means that they are slightly different to those of adults, and so they have their own set of points.

What follows overleaf is a brief treatment for Digestive Blockage in infants. It can be used on children right from birth up to four years of age. Digestive Blockage is not the sole cause of symptoms in children, but this treatment could well do the trick on many a trying occasion! This massage technique can be safely used on children by anyone. As with any complaint, if symptoms persist or worsen or you are in any way worried, contact a health practitioner immediately.

Treatment for Infant Digestive Blockage

1 PUSHING THE SPLEEN CHANNEL

Hold the child's fingers in one hand with their thumb crossing slightly over inwards (see right). Using the outer edge of the end segment of the thumb of your other hand, make a pushing motion along the outer edge of the end segment of the child's thumb. Do this towards the tip of the child's thumb rapidly 100 times to remove blockage from the Spleen, and 100 times the other way to strengthen the Spleen. Your thumb should be at right angles to the direction of movement.

2 PUSHING THE STOMACH CHANNEL

Still holding the child's hand in the same way, do this Pushing technique 100 times on the palm side of the inner section of the child's thumb (see below). This time just push towards the tip of the thumb to reduce blockage in the Stomach.

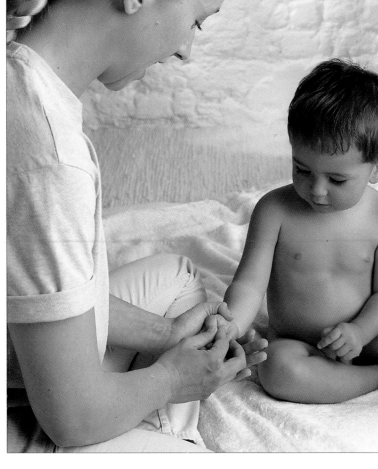

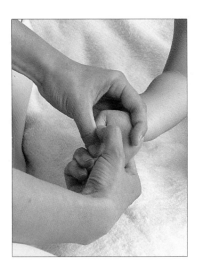

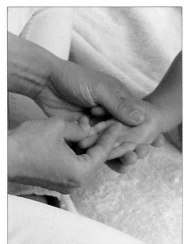

3 PUSHING THE LIVER CHANNEL

Use your thumb and forefinger to hold the child's index finger at the end joint (see left). Use Pushing technique towards the tip of the child's finger to clear the Liver channel. Again, do this 100 times.

4 NIP-KNEADING THE FINGER JOINTS

In this technique, press your thumbnail on to the skin of the first joint of each finger while making the circular motion of Kneading technique (see right). Do this three times on the first joint of all five fingers of each hand in order to open the orifices and clear the flow of digested food.

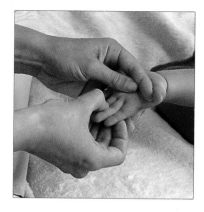

5 STROKING THE BELLY

Using Stroking technique as for adults, work in both clockwise and anticlockwise small circles (following a larger clockwise circle around the circumference of the belly in both instances) to strengthen and unblock the Spleen and Stomach (see below left).

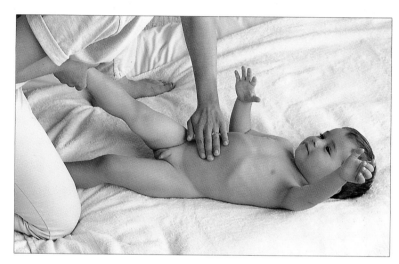

6 KNEADING UB20

Wipe some talcum powder on to the child's spine. Place the middle and index fingers of one hand on to each of the UB20 points (see below); the location is the same as for adults (see page 28). Press downwards – not too hard – while making the circular motion of Kneading technique. This will strengthen and clear the Spleen. To finish, you can apply a small amount of balm to one of the UB20 points to allow the treatment to carry on by itself.

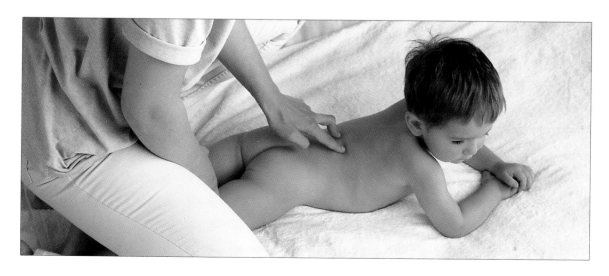

CHAPTER SIX

CHINESE HERBAL MEDICINE

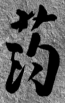

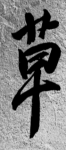

- *The use of herbs in Chinese medicine*
- *Energy and action of herbs*
- *Administration and effect*
- *Herbal medicine as a self-help treatment*
- *Useful herbs and herbal formulae to keep at home*

There are two major methods of treating energetic imbalances available to Chinese medicine: acupuncture and herbal medicines. Traditionally, in China, they are used when other methods such as meditation, dietary changes, exercise and massage have not succeeded. Herbs offer a powerful yet gentle way of helping the body and mind to regain balance, and have, over the centuries, proven to be both safe and effective.

HOW HERBS WORK

Herbs, in the Chinese tradition, include many substances, not just plants; they may be minerals, shells, animals or insects *(see overleaf for further discussion)*. There are over 3,000 substances available to a Chinese herbalist, although most practitioners will stock about 300 herbs for regular use.

The key to understanding the use of Chinese herbs is to realize that they are given from the perspective of energy – Qi and Blood. Each herb has a particular energy which, when matched to the energy of the person, can help restore health. The two essential elements, therefore, are the energy of the person and the energy of the herbs.

This means that the actual herbs used and the exact way in which they are given will vary from case to case according to the needs of the individual.

As you will by now be aware, Chinese medicine generally cools what is hot, and warms what is cold. Herbs are used in this way to rebalance the energies. A diagnosis of the precise energetic balance is an ideal way of ensuring that the correct herbal treatment is applied. However, it is perfectly safe to use the herbs and formulae listed later in this chapter for the symptoms which are mentioned. Make sure that you always follow the guidelines given for their use and adhere to the correct dosage.

HISTORY

Herbal medicine dates right back to the origins of Chinese medicine. The oldest known text dates from 168 BC, 'Formulas for Fifty-two Ailments' (*Wu Shi Er Bing Fang*), and combines herbal formulae with shamanistic practices such as incantations. Once again, this underlines the true origins of Chinese medicine, which are firmly rooted

in beliefs more allied to the alchemists of medieval Europe than to conventional Western scientific thought.

An early collection of formulae was published as the *Shang Han Lun*, 'Discussion of Cold-induced Disorders', by Zhang Zhong Jing around AD 200. This comprehensive collection included over 300 prescriptions

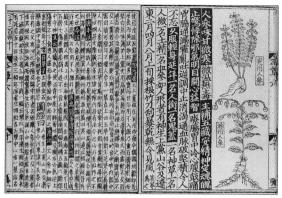

A page from Chongxiu Zhenghe Bencao, *a Chinese herbal text first published in 1802. This shows the entry for ginseng.*

There are various patent formulae included in this chapter, many of which have been in use for centuries. For example, a well-known formula used to treat the digestion, *Bu Zhong Yi Qi Wan* (*see page 118*), was included in 'Discussion of Spleen and Stomach' (*Pi Wei Lun*), written in AD 1249. *Jin Gui Shen Qi Wan* (*see page 120*), which strengthens Kidney Yang, has been in use since at least the second century AD.

Single herbs have also been used for many years; fennel seed, for example, was first mentioned in a text dating back to AD 1061. This long history, along with the gathering of experience over many centuries, testifies to both the effectiveness and the safety of herbal medicine.

that were commonly used at the time, and many of these are still used today (*see page 11 for more on Zhang Zhong Jing*).

ANIMAL PRODUCTS

The use of products derived from living beings may be questioned by people on both ethical and moral grounds. It is also an important consideration for vegetarians and those with certain religious beliefs. I, personally, rarely use products from the animal world, and certainly never if it involves the death of a living being; there are always alternatives which can be used. Some herbs derived from living creatures do not involve death or maltreatment, such as the sloughed-off skin of a cicada (used to treat severe itching in skin disease), which is gathered after the insect has discarded it. It is a feature of this book that *no* products derived from endangered species or living beings are included.

However, it is worth pointing out that there are cultural differences here to be considered. A friend of mine has a father with Parkinson's disease (a disease of the nervous system with stiffness, weakness and shaking). A doctor who had just arrived from China came to see him to recommend treatments. As he was listening to his symptoms, the man's pet tortoise walked across the lawn. The Chinese doctor suggested that he could cook the tortoise and make a soup to drink. The patient was shocked and surprised by the suggestion that he should boil up his pet; the Chinese doctor was, in turn, surprised that there should be any problem with the suggestion.

There has been criticism of Chinese medicine recently in its use of products derived from endangered species, such as tiger bone, bear's gall bladder and rhinoceros horn. This does, sadly, occasionally occur, particularly, but not exclusively, in mainland China. No responsible practitioner would prescribe such items, not least because there are always replacements which can be used instead.

ENERGY AND ACTION OF HERBS

Both herbs and foods have had their energetic actions assessed by experienced practitioners of Chinese medicine. This was done many centuries ago by close observation of individual substances, and their important characteristics were recorded. Such observations were made over many years by physicians of both Taoist and Buddhist traditions. Through meditation and Qi Gong practices, they would observe the effects of taking a single substance and thereby determine its energetic qualities. In this way, through methodical study, the Chinese were able to gather information on plants and their parts — leaves, seeds, flowers, roots, twigs, bark — as well as minerals, shells and parts from the animal world.

There are three things to consider. Firstly, what is the energy of the herb — warming or cooling? Secondly, what is the direction of its energy — ascending or descending? And thirdly, to which organ or part of the body does the energy of the herb pass? These questions indicate the importance that is placed on Qi and its particular characteristics in each herb. In Western science we would want know what *chemicals* a plant contains — its vitamins and minerals. Although this is also useful information, it is Qi that lies at the heart of Chinese medicine; it is Qi that is treated, and it is Qi that is used in treatment, and herbal medicine is no exception. The table below shows a selection of commonly used herbs and their energetic properties, demonstrating just how much the energy and action of different herbs can vary (these herbs are always part of a formula and should not be taken singly).

There are interesting correlations between the part of a plant used and the reason for

REPRESENTATIVE HERBS					
Name	Energy	Taste	Organ affected	Energetic function	Used to treat
Chinese foxglove root (prepared)	Warm	Sweet	Liver, Kidney, Heart	Nourishes Blood and Yin (Water)	Pallor, tiredness and dizziness, night sweats, low back pain
Hoelen	Neutral	Sweet, bland	Heart, Spleen, Lung	Promotes urination, strengthens Spleen, calms Spirit	Oedema, cloudy urine
White atractylodes	Warm	Bitter, sweet	Spleen, Stomach	Strengthens Spleen, dries Dampness	Tiredness, diarrhoea, vomiting
Hawthorn berry	Warm	Sour, sweet	Stomach, Liver	Relieves food stasis, invigorates Blood	Pain in stomach
Gentian	Cold	Bitter	Liver, Gall Bladder, Stomach	Clears Heat, dries Dampness	Jaundice, vaginal discharge, eczema, headache, fever, red eye

its use. The outer parts of the plant such as twigs and leaves tend to work on the outer parts of the body. For example, cinnamon twig is used to treat disorders where Cold and Wind are lodged in the outer levels of the body; this would correspond to the common cold or flu. Roots and tubers which lie deep in the ground are generally used to treat organ problems which lie deep within the body. Minerals and shells such as fossilized bone and oyster shell calm the Spirit. They are heavy and so prevent the Spirit from floating upwards and manifesting as anxiety, dream-disturbed sleep and insomnia.

In addition, herbs which look like a particular body part may be used to treat that area. For example, walnut, which looks like the brain, is used to treat Kidney energy which, according to the principles of Chinese medicine, directly supports and nourishes the brain and mental function. In the West, this idea is already familiar to herbalists and homoeopaths: it is commonly known as the Law of Signatures.

SINGLE HERBS AND FORMULAE

Chinese medicine is generally unique in applying a combination of herbs in treatment, although a single herb can be appropriate in certain circumstances. There are some useful single herbs listed later in this chapter (*see pages 114–117*) and these may be safely used in the home according to the instructions provided (always pay attention to the cautions given for each herb). More often, formulae which contain several herbs mixed together are given. In this way a balanced combination of herbs may be applied to match a person's energy more completely. Formulae are complex combinations of herbs which connect together and interact with each other; such formulae are known as *patents*.

Several herbs together have a stronger effect than a single herb on its own – a synergistic effect. However, combining different herbs also provides for greater safety, as no individual herb which has particularly strong energy or a single action is used in an unprotected manner.

Although formulae are the basis of much of the practice of herbal medicine, they are

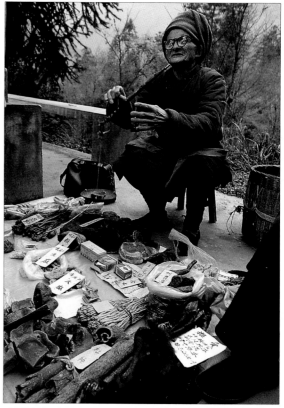

In China, a wide range of herbal products are sold on the street in addition to the hundreds of different herbs and patent formulae stocked by traditional herbal pharmacies.

MODIFYING FORMULAE

Chinese patents can be easily adapted to suit the individual patient.
The illustration below demonstrates how herbs can be added to a
given formulae to treat different symptoms.

LIU WEI DI HUANG WAN
To treat a weakness of the Yin (Water) of the Kidney

     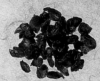

| Chinese foxglove root | Chinese yam | Tree peony root bark | Water plantain tuber | Hoelen | Dogwood fruit |

QI JU DI HUANG WAN
(Herbs added to Liu Wei Di Huang Wan) .
For red or sore eyes

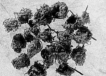 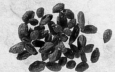

Chrysanthemum flower   Wolfberry

JIN GUI SHEN QI WAN
(Herbs added to Liu Wei Di Huang Wan)
To strengthen Kidney Yang

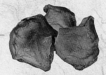 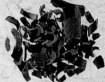

Sichuan aconite root   Cinnamon bark

(Herbs added to Jin Gui Shen Qi Wan)
To strengthen the knees

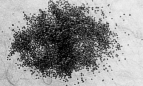

Cuscutae seed

(Herbs added to Jin Gui Shen Qi Wan)
To strengthen the back and alleviate lumbar pain

Eucommia bark   Achyranthes

frequently modified to suit the individual patient. They may be given in different dosages or may have herbs added or omitted depending upon individual requirements. For example, *Liu Wei Di Huang Wan (see page 122)* is a common formula to treat a weakness of the Yin (Water) of the Kidney. If there are associated eye symptoms such as red or sore eyes, chrysanthemum flower and wolfberry are added, and the formula now becomes *Qi Ju Di Huang Wan (see page 122)*. If Kidney Yang is to be treated, then prepared Sichuan aconite root and cinnamon bark are added to *Liu Wei Di Huang Wan* to become *Jin Gui Shen Qi Wan (see page 120)*. In turn, a herb such as cuscutae seed added to *Jin Gui Shen Qi Wan* helps to strengthen the knees, whereas the addition of eucommia bark with achyranthes strengthens the back and also helps to alleviate lumbar pain *(see illustration on previous page)*.

The actions of individual herbs may be modified by preparing them in a particular way. For example: toasting herbs until they are black makes them act more on the Blood; toasting herbs in honey is good if there is any digestive weakness as the sweet taste strengthens the Spleen; and toasting in salt water helps the herb to influence the Kidney.

The above example goes some way towards demonstrating the vast range of options available to a practitioner of herbal medicine with which to address the imbalance correctly, and shows just how specific an individual treatment can be.

APPLICATION AND EFFECTIVENESS

For several years, I only treated people with acupuncture, which is an effective method in many people. However, since I trained in herbal medicine, I have found that I can now treat people with more severe disease both more quickly and more effectively. This is because herbs are strong yet gentle in their action and greatly support the Qi and Blood. They are, essentially, an extension of our diet and so are very nourishing.

In China itself, acupuncture and herbal treatment may be given depending upon the specific cases. In the West, historically, acupuncture developed first, whereas Chinese herbal treatment is a relative latecomer. Today, increasing numbers of people are training in herbal medicine and such treatment is becoming easier to obtain.

There is currently much research being done in China into the effectiveness of herbal medicine. It is used to treat a wide range of conditions, from the common cold to cancer, and from simple anxiety to schizophrenia. Chinese medicine, generally, is recognized to relieve more than fifty specified diseases, including acute infections and chronic degenerative disease.

I have known people who have suffered with symptoms for many years obtain great relief. I once treated a woman who had eczema of the feet, which had caused her problems with walking for over ten years. After taking five bags of herbs, which she boiled up to make a tea, she returned three weeks later, smiling, with a new pair of shoes. Similarly, a woman attended my clinic with a long-standing asthma condition, and after just a month's treatment with herbs, found that her cough, phlegm and wheezing had ceased, never to return.

Although there are a number of different responses to treatment *(see page 154)* and some people take many weeks to improve, such stories reveal the power of Chinese medicine. In my practice, I have found that most people benefit and some enjoy dramatic improvement in their health.

SAFETY AND CONTRA-INDICATIONS

Herbal medicine, along with acupuncture, has to be treated with respect. Of the eight methods of treatment available to Chinese medicine, these two are the strongest and have potentially serious adverse reactions; wrongly applied treatment with both acupuncture and herbs has been known to be fatal. However, the fact that herbal medicine has a long history is some protection and reassurance that it is generally safe.

All the herbs and formulae mentioned in this book are mild and used in low doses. For each, I have listed the symptoms for which they are used; if you pay attention to these and the information given on page 154

about the reactions to treatment (as well as 'Dos and Don'ts' on page 112), the herbs will be perfectly safe.

There is some concern in the West with regard to the toxicity of certain herbs. It is true that there are some individual herbs which have a strong action, and this is why they are not given on their own but are always in a balanced formula. Some herbs are also detoxified by a particular method of preparation, such as soaking in ginger juice.

More serious disease is best treated by properly trained practitioners, and it is their competent practise that will minimize any problems associated with herbal medicine. Guidelines on how to select a practitioner are given on page 149. There are specific occasions when certain herbs and herbal treatments are contra-indicated, or special precautions have to be taken. These are clearly stated in the text.

ADMINISTRATION

There are several different methods of taking herbs, and these vary from country to country and with different practitioners. The most common variations are discussed below.

TEAS

A common method of taking a herbal formula is as a tea. Dried herbs are boiled in water, or a combination of water and wine, for anything up to thirty minutes and the resulting brew sipped. Particular herbs may be added later and boiled for only a brief period of time. Such decoctions have the strongest effect: they are absorbed rapidly, and their effects may even be noticed immediately by some. They are also easy to modify as necessary.

Chinese herbs are of strong Qi, and this can sometimes present difficulties for the Qi of the person, particularly the Stomach Qi. Aversion to the taste of the herbs or nausea may occur for a short time. I find with my patients that although people may dislike the taste at the beginning, this only lasts for a short time. If we are unused to such treatments our stomach may complain for a short time by perceiving the taste as unpleasant.

As treatment progresses, your tastes vary and the herbs become more pleasant. Some people like the taste straight away, so there is a lot of individual variation. If you find that you have continuing problems with taste, other formulations such as pills and capsules may be helpful.

POWDERS

Powders are herbs which have been finely ground. They may be applied to the skin for some skin disorders, or blown into the nose or throat for local effect, or into the nose as in cases of coma. They may also be added to water and boiled, as with decoctions, or infused as with ordinary tea. They are convenient to prepare, can be stored for longer periods and tend to be cheaper. As with decoctions, the taste may present a problem to begin with.

PILLS

Pills are formed from powder and a liquid such as honey, water, rice- or wheat-flour paste or with starch. They are absorbed more slowly and over a longer period of time. They can be stored, are easy to take and tend to be cheaper than dried herbs. They are generally used as tonics for chronic disorders or for acute problems where rapid treatment is needed. Pills are also made if herbs which cannot be boiled are used, as is the case with some very aromatic substances.

SOFT EXTRACTS

Soft extracts are made by simmering herbs with water or vegetable oil, which is then concentrated and turned into a gummy or syrupy consistency. They may be taken internally or used as medicinal plasters.

PATENTS

These are available in several forms including pills, granules, tinctures, oils and liniments, and plasters.

Pills

Pills are primarily manufactured in China and are the equivalent of the pills mentioned above. They are commonly used in China as a convenient method of taking herbs. Standard formulae are available, and these can be obtained from herb shops or are prescribed by herbalists. Western companies also produce such formulae using herbs imported from China; there may be slight modifications to

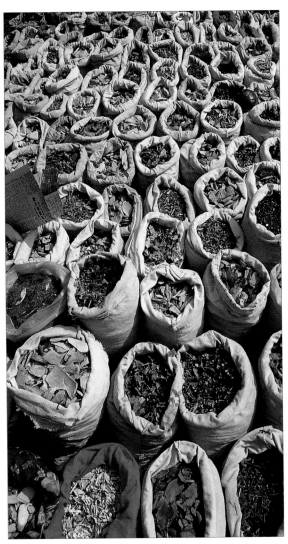

The vast array of herbs available in China in itself underlines the role that herbal medicine commands as an effective and widely used form of treatment.

the formula in the light of experience with Western patients. Patent pills generally work well and many herbalists use them.

There was some controversy a few years ago when it was discovered that some herbal preparations from mainland China for the common cold contained caffeine and paracetamol, and some creams for skin disease contained corticosteroids. These Western drugs were not indicated on the labels. For such reasons it is important to obtain herbs from reputable herb suppliers *(see page 157)*.

Granules

Patent granules are more commonly used in Japan and Taiwan. Large batches of decoctions are boiled, the liquid strained and a dough is made from the residue together with a starch filler. This is made into strands which are then powdered or cut and granules formed. They may be labelled freeze-dried, although this process is never actually used. There are strict rules governing their manufacture in

Japan, and you can be certain that they contain what they claim to contain. Dosages of individual herbs within the formulae may be different to the traditional historical formula.

Tinctures

Patent tinctures have been used in China for thousands of years. They are prepared by soaking the herbs in alcohol, and are used in China mainly for arthritic conditions or occasionally as tonics.

Oils and liniments

These are herbal medicines in the form of an oil-based liquid. They are particularly used for sports injuries and wounds, as they can be rubbed straight on to the affected area.

Plasters

With these, a herbal formula is traditionally applied to material, which is then attached to the skin. This method of application is mainly used for sprains and bruises.

SELF-HELP

There are two ways in which you can help yourself with Chinese herbs. Firstly, there are herbs which can be taken on their own, either for simple problems or regularly for their health-promoting actions. Secondly, there are patents which can be used for specific symptoms to recorrect energetic imbalances. The symptoms listed in chapter seven refer back to these remedies.

I have given the English name for the single herbs and the Chinese 'pinyin' word. When you contact a herbal pharmacy you will need the Chinese word, as this is the exact herb to order. For example, there are two parts of Chinese angelica that are used

in Chinese herbal medicine. They have different actions and are therefore used for different symptoms. *Dang Gui* is the part that is included in this chapter – it is used to strengthen Blood; *Dang Gui Wei* has the action of strongly invigorating Blood – a quite different action. All the patents are known by their Chinese name.

BUILDING A HOME COLLECTION OF BASIC HERBS

In the case of some herbs, it is a simple matter to obtain them because they can be grown in the West, such as sage, or are widely available, such as fresh root ginger. More unusual Chinese herbs may be obtained from a reputable herb supplier, and these are usually found in the major cities in the West. However, you have to be careful when approaching a herbal pharmacy you do not know. It is better to use one that is personally recommended by a qualified herbalist; you will not be able to recognize the herb in many instances, and will certainly not be able to judge its quality.

An important aspect of herbal practice is to ensure that the herbs supplied are what they are claimed to be, and are also of good quality. Sadly, it is sometimes the case that certain suppliers provide herbs which do not fulfil these requirements. The reputable herb suppliers listed at the back of the book provide professional levels of quality control (*see page 157*).

There are several ways in which you can develop a stock of herbal remedies at home. You may be interested in using single herbs for specific first-aid situations or using patent remedies for more general problems.

What to have in your home

The exact herbs and formulae which you might want to keep will depend upon your particular situation. For example, if you live in a damp climate where joint problems and cough are common, you may select the formulae which deal with those. If you are young and generally fit you may have more need for a rubbing oil for sports injuries and remedies for acute colds. For women, the remedies which are more focused on menstruation may be particularly useful. Check through the herbs included in the chart (*see pages 114–125*) and select those which you feel may be helpful. Keep these in a cool, dark cupboard away from children, for use as necessary.

WHAT YOU CAN TREAT YOURSELF AND HOW

Herbs are generally safe but may cause adverse symptoms if they are used for the wrong condition. If you have some Heat inside your body and you take herbs which are heating, you may experience more Heat symptoms, perhaps with feelings of constipation, agitation, insomnia and restlessness, as well as simply feeling hot. Conversely, if you are of a generally cold constitution and you take herbs which are cooling in action, you may find that you experience tiredness, chilly feelings, diarrhoea and water retention.

GUIDELINES FOR USAGE

Do:
- *Follow the dosage indicated, which is for adults unless otherwise shown. Where a range of dosage is shown, begin with the lowest dose and then increase if there is no response. It is generally advisable to consult a professional before you treat children yourself.*
- *Pay heed to the cautions mentioned.*
- *Cook herbs in a glass, stainless steel or earthenware pot (earthenware is the best). Do not use aluminium.*
- *Store any herbal liquid in the refrigerator in a lidded container for up to a week. If you need to take the liquid warm, you can either warm it in a pan or add hot water to the required temperature.*

Don't:
- *Take these herbs long-term (in other words, for several months for a specific symptom). If the symptom recurs when you stop administering the herbs you may not be treating the right symptom, or not treating it at a deep enough level. Seek professional help.*
- *Take herbs if they cause adverse symptoms.*
- *Take herbs unless you are sure that your particular situation is included in the descriptions given in the chart.*

A similar situation to this may arise if you eat cold and raw food.

Herbs may be used safely as self-help for many conditions provided that you are sure they apply to your situation and that you consider the guidelines given in the box below left. (For equivalents to the weights and measures given in the chart overleaf, please see the conversion table below right.)

SINGLE HERBS

As I mentioned earlier, herbs are not commonly used on their own in Chinese medicine; however, there may be occasions when single herbs are helpful. I have selected a small number of single herbs which can be safely used for common symptoms, many of which are already recognizable in the West as they also belong to the tradition of herbalism found there (*see chart on pages 114–117*). Always take heed of the dosages and cautions given for each herb, and pay attention to the guidelines given in the box to the left (it is also helpful to refer to the information on responses of symptoms to treatment given on page 154).

PATENTS

These are standard herbal formulae which have been used over many hundreds of years. There are even archaeological records of some formulae being used in the fourth century BC. Patents usually originate from China, although some herbal companies in the West do produce their own variations based upon an original Chinese formula. Such variations are based upon the experience of treating in a Western environment. There are an increasing number of these, and you can obtain details from the contacts given on page 157. Those I mention here are

Chinese patents and are listed according to their pinyin – Chinese – name (*see chart on pages 118–125*). This is how to order them from a herbal pharmacy. None of those listed here contain animal products. Many of the herbs contained in the patents originate from China, and their names may be quite unfamiliar.

When the dosage is in the form of pills, the number of pills to take is often rather large compared to the dosages associated with Western medicines. Do not be alarmed – this is simply because they are herbal formulae and are gentle in their action. Always take pills with warm water. It is preferable not to treat children or pregnant women without first consulting a practitioner unless it is specifically stated below. Remember to refer to the guidelines given on the previous page and the information on responses of symptoms to treatment on pages 153–154, as well as paying attention to the specific advice on dosage and cautions given for each of the patents.

WEIGHTS AND MEASURES

Certain weights and measures are used in reference to instructions for use for the herbs featured in the charts on the following pages. For the appropriate conversions, please refer to the list given below:

- *2.5 cm = 1 inch*
- *1 teaspoon = 5 ml*
- *3 teaspoons = 1 tablespoon = 15 ml*
- *2 tablespoons = 1 fl oz = 30 ml*
- *1 cup = 8 fl oz = 0.24 litre*
- *2 cups = 1 pint = 0.47 litre*
- *4 cups = 1 quart = 0.95 litre*
- *28 g = 1 oz*

SINGLE HERBS	Energy	Energetic action	Organs	
Black Pepper (*Hu Jiao*)	Hot, spicy (pungent)	Warms Stomach and disperses Cold	Stomach, Large Intestine	
Cardamom (*Sha Ren*)	Warm, spicy (pungent), aromatic	Moves Qi, strengthens Stomach, transforms Dampness and stops vomiting	Spleen, Stomach	
Chinese Angelica (*Dang Gui*)	Warm	Nourishes the Blood and moistens the Intestines	Heart, Liver	
Chrysanthemum Flower (*Ju Hua*)	Cool	Disperses Wind, clears Heat and brightens the eyes	Lung, Liver	
Cinnamon Bark (*Rou Gui* and *Gui Pi*)	*Cinnamon comes in several forms. The best quality is* Rou Gui *which can be obtained from a Chinese herbal pharmacy; top grade cinnamon bark comes in the form of the bark itself and is very expensive.* Gui Pi *is of a lesser quality but cheaper, and adequate for most purposes. Powdered cinnamon and cinnamon sticks are satisfactory but of lower quality than* Gui Pi.			
	Hot	Warms Kidneys, strengthens Yang, warms Stomach and warms all the Channels	Kidneys, Spleen, Liver, Urinary Bladder	
Cloves (*Ding Xiang*)	Warm	Warms Stomach	Stomach, Spleen, Kidney	
Coltsfoot (*Tian Hua Fen*)	Sweet, cold	Transforms Hot Phlegm	Lung, Stomach, Large Intestine	
Fennel Seed (*Xiao Hui Xiang*)	Warm	Warms Stomach and moves Liver Qi	Stomach, Liver	

Used to treat	How to use	Cautions
Vomiting and sore throat due to Cold invasion	Grate a I cm piece of fresh root ginger and grind five black peppercorns, and bring to the boil in 2 cups of water. Simmer until the liquid has reduced by two thirds. Strain, and drink warm in three doses through the day.	Do not use if there are night sweats or other signs of Heat such as mouth ulcers, burning pain or hot feelings in the body.
Nausea, vomiting, diarrhoea and abdominal pain	To make a tea, add boiling water to the ground seeds of six pods of cardamom. Drink when warm.	Do not use if there are night sweats or other signs of Heat such as mouth ulcers, burning pain or hot feelings in the body.
Anaemia, pallor with tiredness, palpitations, floaters in the vision and insomnia	Use in a soup to nourish the Blood (see recipe on page 60).	Do not use if there are loose stools, poor appetite, indigestion or night sweats.
Sore, red and dry eyes	Boil six flower heads in I cup of water for two minutes. Strain off the liquid and allow to cool. Bathe eyes in the cool liquid or wipe with soaked cotton wool. Alternatively, pour I cup of hot water on to I teaspoon of the dried herb (2 teaspoons fresh herb). Leave for five minutes and strain. Bathe eyes as above.	Seek professional help if symptoms do not subside within a few days of use.
Impotence, cold and weakness in the lower back and legs, nausea, vomiting and diarrhoea due to Cold in the Stomach, and for painful periods when the pain begins just before menstruation	Make a tea by pouring boiling water on to a 2–3 cm piece of cinnamon stick or half a level teaspoon of powdered bark. Drink when warm. Chew a small piece of the bark after exposure to cold to prevent subsequent invasion of Cold leading to common cold or flu.	Do not use during pregnancy, or if there are night sweats or other signs of Heat such as mouth ulcers, burning pain or hot feelings in the body.
Nausea, vomiting due to Cold in the Stomach, hiccups due to weakness of Stomach Qi, impotence, flatulence and vaginal discharge due to weakness of Kidney Yang	Add four cloves to stir-fried vegetables, with cardamom and ginger to warm the Stomach. May also be added to baked or stewed fruit. Grind cloves before use, or remove before eating. To make a tea add 2–4 g cloves and a I cm piece of grated fresh root ginger to 2 cups of water; simmer until liquid reduces to I cup. Drink half a cup, warm, daily for nausea and vomiting. To relieve flatulence, pour I cup of hot water on to five or six cloves; steep for five minutes and drink when warm.	Cautions: Do not use if there are night sweats or other signs of Heat such as mouth ulcers, burning pain or hot feelings in the body.
Cough with thick, yellow sputum	Make a tea by soaking I tablespoon of dried coltsfoot flower in 4 cups of cold water for a few minutes. Bring to the boil and simmer for twenty minutes. Drink the warm liquid in three equal doses.	Do not use in cases of diarrhoea or if there are cold feelings.
Nausea, vomiting and headache due to Cold in the Stomach, abdominal pain due to Cold, digestive upsets and painful periods. It can also be used to aid the flow of milk when breast-feeding	Make a tea using I teaspoon of seeds (or 5–8 cm of fennel stalk cut into small pieces). Place in a mug and add boiling water; drink when warm. This is good for digestive upsets. Add cinnamon bark as above for lower abdominal pain with feelings of coldness or for painful menstruation at the start of, or prior to, the period. To help flow of milk, boil I teaspoon of seeds in barley water and drink the liquid when warm.	Do not use if there are night sweats or other signs of Heat such as mouth ulcers, burning pain or hot feelings in the body.

SINGLE HERBS	Energy	Energetic action	Organs	
Ginger, fresh root (*Sheng Jiang*)	*Use only the fresh root. Dried ginger is much hotter in nature and is indicated for different situations completely. Some ginger sold in health food shops is of the dried variety.*			
	Warm	Warms Stomach and disperses Cold	Lungs, Stomach	
Ginseng root (*Ren Shen*)	*This is strong in action and generally given as part of a formula, but can also be helpful when used singly. There are three types of ginseng: Chinese, Korean and American. They have different energetic properties. Chinese ginseng, the one used here, mainly affects the Lungs and Heart and is used to strengthen Qi. Asiabell root (Dang Shen) is often substituted as it is cheaper yet has similar functions.*			
	Warm	Strengthens Qi, benefits Yin, generates fluids and calms the Spirit	Spleen, Lung	
Liquorice (*Gan Cao*)	*This is a common constituent of many formulae as it balances the actions of other herbs, but it also has beneficial effects when used on its own. It harmonizes the digestion and so may be used for the apparently contradictory symptoms of diarrhoea and constipation.*			
	Neutral (warm if toasted in honey)	Strengthens Qi, moistens Lungs, stops coughing, clears Heat and acts as an antidote to toxins	All organs, but particularly the Spleen and Lung	
Mint (*Bo He*)	Cool	Disperses WindHeat, helps the throat, smooths Liver Qi, and clears the head and eyes	Lung, Liver	
Polygonum root (*He Shou Wu*)	*The Chinese name is translated as 'Black Haired Mr He'. The story is that a man with white hair took this herb and his hair became black.*			
	Warm	Nourishes Blood, strengthens Kidneys and Jing (Kidney function is related to health of head hair) and moistens the Intestines	Liver, Kidneys	
Sage (*Dan Shen*)	*Use the leaves as they are more readily available than the root (Dan Shen). The information here about energies and organs refers to the root, which is not generally used on its own. The leaves are quite safe to use as detailed under 'How to use' and will be a useful addition to your herbal pharmacy.*			
	Cold, bitter	Moves the Blood and clears Heat	Heart, Pericardium, Liver	

Used to treat	How to use	Cautions
Nausea, vomiting, indigestion and headache caused by eating cold foods, cough, common cold, symptoms after exposure to cold and dampness	To make a tea, grate a 1 cm piece of peeled fresh root ginger into a mug; add boiling water and leave for five minutes. Add a teaspoon of honey and drink when warm. For the common cold or exposure to cold, add a squeeze of lemon and a tot of whiskey. To warm the Stomach and aid the digestion, use grated in soups and stir-fried foods or add to fruit and then bake or stew to warm the energy of the fruit.	Do not use if there is excess thirst, mouth ulcers, burning sensation in the upper abdomen or coughing of yellow or green sputum.
Poor appetite, tiredness, diarrhoea, excessive sweating, impotence and frequent urination	Add 5 g of ginseng to 2 cups of water and boil down to 1 cup. Drink this liquid, warm, in three doses throughout the day.	Do not use if there is high blood pressure or if there are night sweats or other signs of Heat such as mouth ulcers, burning pain or hot feelings in the body. Long-term or inappropriate use may lead to feelings of heat in the chest, night sweats, anxiety and palpitations.
Poor appetite, tiredness and diarrhoea caused by weakness of Spleen Qi, indigestion, constipation, cough, sore throat and fever	Either chew the raw root or make a tea by adding boiling water to 10 g of the raw herb. Drink the liquid when warm. For constipation boil 80 g in 4 cups of water and simmer for ten minutes. Allow to cool and drink a cupful two or three times a day.	Do not use when there is nausea, vomiting or excess Dampness (mucus) in the body, or if there is water retention or high blood pressure.
Acute fever with headache and cough, sore throat, pre-menstrual syndrome with irritability, sore breasts and headache	Make a tea by adding boiling water to three bruised or crushed leaves of fresh mint (half a teaspoon of dried mint). Add a teaspoon of honey and drink when warm. For treatment of mastitis in breast-feeding mothers, soak 1 tablespoon of dried leaves in 4 cups of water for a few minutes. Bring to the boil and simmer for twenty minutes. Strain and soak a cloth in the liquid when warm, then apply to the breast.	Do not use if there are night sweats. Long-term daily use will weaken the Qi. If symptoms do not subside seek professional help.
Anaemia, weak back and knees, dizziness, floaters in the vision, pallor and tiredness	Soak 1 tablespoon of the dried herb in 4 cups of water for a few minutes. Bring to the boil and simmer for twenty minutes. Drink one quarter of a cup, warm, twice daily before meals.	Do not use if there is poor appetite, diarrhoea, excess mucus in throat or cough with sputum.
Cough and cold associated with fever, sore throat and mouth ulcers. It can also be used externally for bruises	To make a tea, pour 1 cup of hot water on to 1 teaspoon of the dried herb (2 teaspoons of the fresh herb), leave for five minutes, strain and drink when warm. This is good for cough and common cold associated with headache and fever. Apply externally for bruises. To relieve a sore throat, soak 1 tablespoon of dried sage in 4 cups of cold water. Simmer for twenty minutes, strain and gargle with the warm liquid. For sore gums and mouth ulcers, use the warm liquid as a mouthwash.	Do not use if there is weakness and tiredness with pallor and dizziness.

PATENTS	Contents	Energetic Action	
An Mian Pian	Sour jujube, Chinese senega root, gardenia fruit, hoelen and liquorice	Cools Heat in the Liver and calms the mind	
Ba Zhen Wan	*This is translated as 'Women's Precious Pills' because it is a common formula given to women. It is a frequently used Qi and Blood tonic containing four herbs to strengthen each.*		
	Ginseng or Asiabell root, hoelen, white atractylodes, Chinese angelica, Sichuan lovage root, Chinese foxglove root, white peony root and liquorice	Strengthens Qi and nourishes Blood	
Bi Yan Pian	Xanthium fruit, magnolia flower, amur cork-tree bark, liquorice, Chinese angelica, forsythia fruit, schizandra fruit, balloonflower root, anemarrhena root, chrysanthemum flower, ledebouriella root and schizonepeta stem/bud	Resolves Phlegm and Dampness particularly affecting the head and nose	
Bu Zhong Yi Qi Wan	Ginseng or Asiabell root, white atractylodes, yellow milk-vetch, Chinese angelica, tangerine peel, Hare's ear root, black cohosh rhizome, liquorice, fresh ginger and black date	Strengthens and raises Spleen Qi	
Chuan Bei Jing Pian	Liquorice, tangerine peel, schizandra fruit, Chinese senega root, fritillary bulb and balloonflower root	Removes Phlegm from the Lungs and relieves cough	
Chuan Bei Pi Pa Gao	Fritillary bulb, loquat leaf, beech silver-toproot, honey, balloonflower root, apricot seed, mint, tussilago, prepared pinellia rhizome, tangerine peel and schizandra fruit	Moistens the Lungs, clears Heat and relieves cough	
Chuan Bei Pi Pa Lu	Fritillary bulb, stemona root, mint, loquat leaf and sweet tasting flavouring to make a syrup	Clears Heat from the Lungs and transforms Phlegm	
Dang Gui Pian	Chinese angelica, Sichuan lovage root, white atractylodes and red Chinese date	Nourishes the Blood and strengthens Spleen Qi	
Die Da Wan Hua You	*This is a rubbing oil traditionally used for cuts and bruises sustained during martial arts.*		
	Drynaria root, safflower flower, aloeswood, chimonanthus flower, pyrolusitum, myrrh, frankincense, dragon's blood resin (a plant) and pseudoginseng root	Helps blood circulation, reduces swelling, relaxes muscles and relieves pain	
Ding Xin Wan	*This is a variant of* Gui Pi Wan *but the modifications make it more suitable for insomnia.*		
	Arbor-vitae seed, Chinese angelica, hoelen, Chinese senega root, sour jujube, creeping lily-turf tuber, Asiabell root, skullcap root and amber	Strengthens Qi, nourishes Blood and calms the mind	

Used to treat	Dosage	Cautions
Insomnia associated with anxiety, dream-disturbed sleep, red and sore eyes and irritability	4 pills three times daily	Do not use long-term.
Tiredness, pallor, dizziness, shortness of breath, floaters in the vision, palpitations, anxiety, heavy menstruation with feelings of tiredness during or after the period, and weakness after childbirth	8–10 pills three times daily	Do not use in the first two weeks after childbirth or if there is poor appetite, loose stools or indigestion.
Blocked nose, runny nose and hay fever	5 pills four times daily	Do not use long-term.
Tiredness, poor appetite, loose stools, prolapse and heavy menstrual bleeding	8 pills three times daily	Do not use during pregnancy or if there are headaches, symptoms of Heat/night sweats, or if there is Damp accumulation (see page 36).
Cough with sputum which is white and profuse or sticky	3–6 pills three times daily	Do not use for the first stages of a cold or if there is a fever.
Cough which is dry with little or no sputum as the Heat has dried the sputum. There may also be fever and dryness of mouth and throat	2 teaspoons three times a day. Children over five can be given 1 teaspoon three times daily (add to warm water)	Do not use for cough with sputum.
Cough with thick yellow sputum, dry throat with thirst and sore throat	2–3 teaspoons three to four times daily. Children under five take one third of dose; under twelves take half of dose	Do not use for cough with white sputum.
Weakness and tiredness, particularly after childbirth or due to heavy periods	5 pills three times daily	Do not use in first two weeks after childbirth, or if there is poor appetite, loose stools or indigestion.
Sports injuries, sprains or strains and open wounds	Rub on to affected area three times daily. For open wounds, soak lint or dressing with oil, apply and bandage. Renew daily	Keep away from eyes and wash hands after use.
Insomnia associated with palpitations, anxiety, tiredness and poor memory	6 pills twice daily	Do not use long-term.

PATENTS	Contents	Energetic Action	
Du Huo Ji Sheng Wan	*This is a famous formula for long-standing joint pains with weakness of Qi and Blood.*		
	Pubescent angelica root, large-leaf gentian root, ledebouriella root, wild ginger, mulberry mistletoe stem, eucommia bark, achyranthes root, cinnamon bark, Chinese angelica, Sichuan lovage root, cooked Chinese foxglove root, white peony root, ginseng or Asiabell root, hoelen and liquorice	Moves Qi and Blood in the muscles and joints, strengthens the Qi and nourishes the Blood	
Er Chen Wan	*This formula clears mucus out of the body. It does not contain herbs which strengthen the Qi, and so should not be taken long-term, particularly in a cold and damp climate.*		
	Prepared pinellia rhizome, tangerine peel, liquorice and hoelen	Moves Qi and transforms Dampness and Phlegm	
Gui Pi Wan	*This is a common formula for women who have heavy blood loss during a period and associated emotional symptoms. It is often prescribed for problems around the menopause.*		
	Ginseng or Asiabell root, hoelen, yellow milk-vetch, white atractylodes, sour jujube, Chinese senega root, Chinese angelica, costus root, longan fruit, liquorice, black date and fresh ginger	Strengthens the Spleen Qi and nourishes the Heart Blood	
Jin Gui Shen Qi Wan	*This is also known as Kidney Qi pill or Rehmannia Eight, and is Liu Wei Di Huang Wan with the addition of cinnamon bark and prepared Sichuan aconite root. There may be a substitution for prepared Sichuan aconite root depending upon the source.*		
	Chinese foxglove root, dogwood fruit, Chinese yam, tree peony root bark, water plantain tuber, hoelen, cinnamon bark and prepared Sichuan aconite root	Strengthens Kidney Yang	
Liu Jun Zi Wan	*This is translated as 'Six Gentlemen Pills' because it usually contains six herbs to strengthen the Spleen and resolve Dampness.*		
	Ginseng or Asiabell root, white atractylodes, hoelen, tangerine peel, liquorice, prepared pinellia rhizome, fresh ginger and black date	Similar to *Er Chen Wan* (*see above*) but also strengthens Lung and Spleen Qi	
Liu Wei Di Huang Wan	*This is also known as Rehmannia Six — an ancient formula and the basis for several others.*		
	Chinese foxglove root, dogwood fruit, Chinese yam, tree peony root bark, hoelen and water plantain tuber	Nourishes the Yin of the Kidney and Liver	
Ping Wei Pian	White atractylodes, tangerine peel, liquorice and magnolia bark	Calms Stomach, resolves Dampness and strengthens the Spleen and Stomach	

Used to treat	Dosage	Cautions
Joint pains, pain in lower back and knees with coldness	9 pills twice daily	Do not use for hot and red joints of recent onset.
Cough with profuse white sputum, cotton-wool feeling in the head, nausea, and perhaps vomiting of mucus	8 pills three times daily or 2 honey pills twice daily	Do not use if you feel excessively tired, have diarrhoea or are in a cold climate. In such cases you may be better with *Liu Jun Zi Wan (see below)*.
Poor appetite, anxiety, palpitations, tiredness and perhaps insomnia or waking in the night	8 pills three times daily	This is a safe formula. Use according to the guidelines on page 112.
Impotence, low back pain with cold feelings, weak knees, frequent urination, cough, fluid retention and diarrhoea, particularly early in the morning	8–10 pills three times daily	Do not use if there are symptoms of Heat or night sweats, or during pregnancy.
Tiredness, loose stools and poor appetite, plus symptoms listed under *Er Chen Wan*	8 pills three times daily	Do not use if there are symptoms of Heat or night sweats.
Tinnitus, deafness, night sweating, difficult urination and low back ache. This is Kidney weakness associated with Heat symptoms. Compare with those under *Jin Gui Shen Qi Wan*, which treats Kidney weakness with cold symptoms	8–16 pills three times daily	Do not use if there is poor appetite, loose stools or indigestion.
Poor appetite, loose stools, nausea, indigestion and abdominal bloating	4 pills twice daily	Do not use long-term.

PATENTS	Contents	Energetic Action	
Qi Ju Di Huang Wan	*This is Liu Wei Di Huang Wan with wolfberry and chrysanthemum flower added.*		
	Chinese foxglove root, dogwood fruit, Chinese yam, tree peony root bark, hoelen, water plantain tuber, wolfberry and chrysanthemum flower	Nourishes the Yin of the Kidney and Liver, soothes the eyes and calms Wind	
Qian Lie Xian Wan	Cow soapwort seed, tree peony root bark, red peony root, hogfennel root, liquorice, costus root, akebia stem, yellow milk-vetch root and patrinia.	Clears DampHeat from the pelvis and aids the circulation of Blood	
Qing Qi Hua Tan Wan	Prepared pinellia rhizome, Jack-in-the-pulpit, snakegourd root, scutellaria, tangerine peel, apricot seed and hoelen	Clears PhlegmHeat in the Lungs	
Ren Dan	Liquorice, balloonflower root, white or black cutch, cardamom, camphor, mint, cloves and borneol	Clears Summer-heat and regulates Stomach and Spleen	
Ren Shen Yang Rong Wan	Ginseng, white atractylodes, yellow milk-vetch root, tangerine peel, Chinese foxglove root, schizandra fruit, hoelen, black date, white peony root, Chinese senega root, cinnamon bark, fresh ginger and liquorice	Strengthens Qi and Blood, with a particular emphasis on Blood and the Yang of the Spleen and Kidney	
Run Chang Wan	*This contains cannabis seed, which moistens the Intestines and so is helpful for constipation due to Dryness. When given as a dried herb, it is always cooked so that it cannot be grown.*		
	Cannabis seed, peach seed, notopterygium root, Chinese angelica and rhubarb	Clears Heat, moistens the Intestines and aids defecation	
Sang Ju Yin	Mulberry leaf, balloonflower root, apricot seed, reed rhizome, forsythia fruit, chrysanthemum flower, mint and liquorice	Disperses Wind and Heat attacking the Lungs	
Shen Chu Cha	Magnolia bark, balloonflower root, pubescent angelica root, sweet wormwood, Chinese yam, amber, hoelen, wheat chaff, cardamom, scutellaria, immature bitter orange fruit, notopterygium root and quince	Calms the Stomach, resolves Phlegm and settles the digestion	
Shi Chuan Da Bu Wan	*This formula is similar to Ren Shen Yang Rong Wan, which mainly strengthens Qi and Blood, but particularly Blood.*		
	Ginseng or Asiabell root, yellow milk-vetch root, white peony root, white atractylodes, hoelen, Chinese foxglove root, Chinese angelica, cinnamon bark, Sichuan lovage root and liquorice	Strengthens Qi and Blood, but particularly Qi	

Used to treat	Dosage	Cautions
Red and sore eyes, in addition to the symptoms listed under *Liu Wei Di Huang Wan*	8 pills three times daily	Do not use if there is poor appetite, loose stools or indigestion.
Cystitis with low back and abdominal pain	6 pills three times daily	Stop using as soon as symptoms have disappeared.
Cough with yellow, sticky sputum	6 pills three times daily	Do not use for first stages of a common cold or for dry cough.
Symptoms after being exposed to very hot sun, such as diarrhoea, sunstroke, heat exhaustion and travel sickness	30–60 pellets twice daily. Children over five take 10 pellets each dose	Do not use if there are symptoms of Cold.
Tiredness, poor appetite, low back ache, and when generally feeling run down	6 pills three times daily or 1 honey pill twice daily	This is a safe formula. Use according to the guidelines on page 112.
Constipation due to Heat; look for associated symptoms of dry, 'bitty' stools, thirst, restlessness, agitation and night sweats	4 pills three times daily	Do not use for constipation with feelings of Cold.
First few days of a common cold with symptoms of dry and sore throat, fever, headache, dry cough, runny nose and watering eyes	4 pills two to four times daily	Do not use long-term.
Belching, loose stools, abdominal bloating and nausea. This range of symptoms is caused by an accumulation of Phlegm or food stuck in the Stomach	Take one block (compressed dried herbs) twice daily. Place in cup and add boiling water; drink when warm	Do not use for diarrhoea with tiredness and feelings of Cold.
Tiredness, pallor, cold limbs, palpitations, dizziness and insomnia	8 pills three times daily	Do not use if there are symptoms of Heat in the body such as night sweats, mouth ulcers or feelings of heat.

PATENTS	Contents	Energetic Action	
Shu Gan Wan	*This formula's emphasis is on the Stomach and it is somewhat similar in its action to Xiao Yao Wan, which concentrates more on the Liver.*		
	Sichuan Chinaberry fruit, aloeswood, corydalis tuber, costus root, white peony root, hoelen, immature bitter orange fruit, tangerine peel, cardamom, magnolia bark and turmeric tuber	Smooths Liver Qi which is attacking the Stomach	
Tian Wan Bu Xin Dan	*This is known as 'Celestial Emperor Heart-supplementing Elixir', in reference to the Heart as the Emperor that rules through its connection with heaven. The Heart is the most important organ in the body as it houses the mind, and so is connected with matters of the Spirit (heaven).*		
	Raw Chinese foxglove root, creeping lily-turf tuber, ziziphus seed, arbor-vitae seed, schizandra fruit, Chinese angelica, asparagus, figwort root, sage root, balloonflower root, Chinese senega root and hoelen	Strengthens Yin, clears Heat, strengthens the Heart and calms the Spirit	
Xiang Sha Yang Wei Pian	White atractylodes, cardamom, costus root, sprouted barley, tangerine peel, liquorice, Asiabell root and medicated leaven	Strengthens the Spleen and Stomach	
Xiao Yao Wan	*This formula is translated as 'Relaxed Wanderer', as it gently allows Liver Qi to move. Its energy is often described as being similar to that of the early morning when the dew is on the ground, the first light of the sun gently shines through the trees and all is quiet and peaceful.*		
	Bupleurum, Chinese angelica, white atractylodes, white peony root, hoelen, liquorice, fresh ginger and mint	Smooths the flow of Liver Qi	
Yang Yin Qing Fei Tan	Tree peony root bark, fritillary bulb, white peony root, figwort root, raw Chinese foxglove root, creeping lily-turf tuber, liquorice and mint	Nourishes Lung Yin	
Yao Tong Pian	Chinese angelica, dipsacus root, wolfberry fruit, white atractylodes, scurfy pea fruit, achyranthes root and eucommia bark	Strengthens the Kidneys and moves Qi and Blood in the lower back	
Yin Qiao Jie Du Pian	*These may also be known simply as* Yin Qiao *pills.*		
	Honeysuckle flower, forsythia fruit, balloonflower root, mint and schizonepeta stem/bud	Disperses Wind and Heat invasion	
Yu Dai Wan	Cooked Chinese foxglove root, Chinese angelica, white peony root, amur cork-tree bark, Sichuan lovage root, Tree of Heaven bark and black cardamom fruit	Clears DampHeat in the pelvis	

Used to treat	How to use	Cautions
Nausea, belching, vomiting, acid regurgitation, full feelings in the stomach and indigestion after eating	8 pills three times daily	Do not use long-term.
Insomnia, palpitations, restlessness, agitation, poor memory and concentration. In more severe cases there may be ulcers on the tongue or mouth; there may also be Heat signs such as night sweats	8 pills three times daily	Do not use long-term.
Weaker people with indigestion, heartburn, poor appetite, belching, nausea, loose stools and tiredness	4 pills three times daily	Do not use long-term.
Headaches, pre-menstrual syndrome, breast soreness, irritability, belching, indigestion and inability to fall asleep at night	8 pills three times daily	Do not use during pregnancy.
Dry cough or cough with scanty sputum, sore and dry throat. It is particularly useful for a dry cough which persists after a common cold has subsided	4 teaspoons twice daily	Do not use for cough with sputum.
Low backache with an underlying Kidney Yang weakness	6 pills three times daily or 1 honey pill three times daily	Do not use long-term.
First stage of a common cold or flu; sudden onset of aversion to cold, fever, headache with perhaps a sore throat and cough	5–6 pills every three hours. After three doses, take every six hours as needed. Do not take beyond the third day after symptoms began	Some formulations contain Western drugs; always check the label. One variation contains antelope horn. Ask for those manufactured in Beijing.
Yellow vaginal discharge often accompanied by lower abdominal pain, burning urination and itching	8 pills three times daily	Do not use for white vaginal discharge.

CHAPTER SEVEN

SELF-HELP FOR COMMON SYMPTOMS

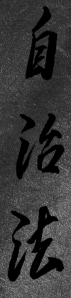

- *Using Chinese medicine to treat symptoms at home*
- *Comprehensive chart of common symptoms listing methods of treatment*
- *When to seek professional help*

One of the main purposes of this book is to show you how you can help to relieve discomfort and other specific symptoms using Chinese medicine. This chapter includes a wide range of common symptoms, all of which are cross-referenced to the advice on diet, massage and herbal medicine in previous chapters. For maximum clarity and ease of reference, this information is presented in a chart to give you a complete view of the methods available to treat each symptom.

USING THE COMMON-SYMPTOMS CHART

In the chart I refer to names of symptoms rather than 'disease labels', because people talk in terms of how they feel. Consequently, this section is accessible and practical without being too 'medical'. This book is not intended to teach you how to self-diagnose but rather how to become aware of certain symptoms, learn how to understand them in terms of Chinese medicine and apply simple remedies based on the methods given.

The symptoms featured in the chart are commonly seen. They are described from the perspective of Chinese medicine and treatments are given which can help relieve them. When you consult a particular symptom, you may find it helpful to refer to the information in chapter two. This will refresh your memory and enable you to understand the underlying energetic imbalance, especially when a disturbance of a particular organ is mentioned.

Meditation and Qi Gong are excellent practices to maintain health and strengthen us in general. I would encourage you to practise them regularly, whatever your level of health, and thus they are only mentioned in the chart when they are of particular importance.

The information on diet emphasizes what is considered to be a healthy way of eating, and advises which foods to eat more of and those to avoid.

Massage is a major aspect of any self-help programme; review the information about massage media on page 89 and keep at least one of these at home. Begin gently – remember that you are working with Qi and strong force is not necessary.

Herbal medicine is also effective in relieving symptoms. Both single herbs and patent formulae are given as treatments. If there is a choice of herbs to take, refer to chapter six to decide which one is most suitable. Always pay attention to the guidelines listed on page 112.

WHEN TO SEEK HELP
Self-help can be applied safely and effectively in many situations. This is certainly true of all the suggested methods of treatment for the symptoms included in the chart. There are times, though, when professional help is necessary, such as for severe acute illness. Advice on when to seek professional help is given for each symptom, but if you are in any doubt about your condition consult a practitioner.

SYMPTOM

Anxiety

This is a common state of inner tension; generally, there are feelings of anxiety, nervousness, apprehension or anticipation and, in some cases, panic. There can be poor concentration, indecision, restlessness and agitation. Sleep may be disturbed, either with difficulty going to sleep or waking in the night; dreams can be vivid. Severe attacks may be accompanied by shortness of breath with feelings of faintness (hyperventilation). Meditation is very helpful for anxiety; try the breathing relaxation on page 51 before going on to the specific meditations. As you practise, your mind will calm and settle; with perseverance you will experience highly beneficial effects.

Some cases are due to a weakness of Qi and Blood. Here there will be associated symptoms of pallor, tiredness, blurred or weak vision with floaters, dizziness and perhaps shortness of breath. There may be dream-disturbed sleep, insomnia and anxiety as the mind is not grounded and nourished adequately. If insomnia is a particular feature, refer to that specific symptom on page 140.

Other cases may be due to Phlegm and Heat interrupting the function of the Heart. The Heart houses the mind, and consequently becomes unsettled. Associated symptoms include irritability, dream-disturbed sleep, restlessness and perhaps night sweats. If insomnia is a particular feature refer to that specific symptom on page 140.

Backache

This is a common symptom and many thousands of working hours are lost each year due to consequent limitation of activity. Not only is this a great economic loss but, more importantly, people suffer back pain which limits them in their lives. The pain may come on suddenly and be severe but, more often, it is long-standing and comes on recurrently. The site of the pain may be an indication of underlying organ problems which may be present. If you refer to the illustration in chapter two (*see page 28*), you will see the position of the points on the back (known as Back Transporting Points) which refer to the organs mentioned below. Imbalance in these organs will give pain at the level of the associated point.

Pain in the lower back is related to the function of the Kidney, pain in the lower chest area at the back related to Liver, Stomach or Spleen problems and pain in the upper chest area at the back related to a Heart or Lung problem. Pain in the upper back and neck area can be related to Gall Bladder problems and its paired organ, the Liver.

Meditation and Qi Gong are particularly helpful for strengthening the Kidneys as they are deeply nourishing. Begin with general breathing relaxation and then go on

LOWER BACK AND GENERAL
There may be an invasion of a climatic factor such as wind, cold or dampness. This is common in manual workers who work outside and become cold or wet. The onset of the pain is sudden and tends to be severe. The painful area may feel cold and is stiff. There is not usually any great degree of an organ imbalance, although you should consider this if the backache is recurrent or associated with other symptoms. Acupuncture treatment by a professional is extremely effective for such problems and may get rid of acute pain in one treatment, but there are also a number of treatments you can apply at home.

LOWER BACK
A more common cause of low back pain, and one which is certainly the case in long-standing, recurrent problems, is a weakness of the energy of the Kidney. There may associated symptoms of frequency of urination, weak knees, tiredness, impotence and vaginal discharge.

NECK AND SHOULDERS
Pain and stiffness in the neck and shoulders is often associated with obstruction to the smooth flow of Liver Qi; emotional stress and tension therefore plays a large part. You may also find it helpful to refer to pain and stiffness in the joints on page 144.

TREATMENT

Diet	Massage	Herbs	Seek professional help
A generally healthy diet (*see page 59*) with foods which benefit the Qi and Yang and those which help strengthen the Blood and Yin (*see page 55*).	Knead points UB15, UB17, UB20, UB21 on the back (*see pages 91 and 95*). Alternatively, do Vibrating on CV6, CV14, H7 and P6 with St37 (*see page 98*). You may select either group of points for a treatment (*see pages 26–28 for points*).	*Gui Pi Wan* for most cases (*see page 120*). In more severe situations of anxiety it may be helpful to begin with *Tian Wan Bu Xin Dan* (*see page 124*).	• If symptoms are severe • If there are mental symptoms, such as hallucinations and delusions
A generally healthy diet (*see page 59*) with foods that help resolve Dampness (*see page 55*). Avoid foods with very hot energy, such as chilli, cayenne, paprika, coffee, alcohol and greasy food. Also, reduce or avoid foods which generate Dampness (*see page 55*).	Knead points UB15, CV14, H7, P6 with GB34 and St40 (*see pages 91 and 95 for Kneading technique, and pages 26–28 for points*).		
	Treat UB23, UB40 and GV26 for the lower back (*see pages 26–28 for points*). Use local points for acute back pain in other areas. These will be tender, feel tense to the touch, may be warm, cold or slightly discoloured: they are known as *Ah Shi* points. Massage to these will release the obstruction to Qi and Blood and allow healing to take place. The massage will be uncomfortable and should be repeated regularly to disperse the congested areas. Do Kneading on all points (*see pages 91 and 95*), and lateral Burnishing technique (*see page 94*) on UB23 and UB40.	Use a ginger compress; the heat of the compress and the warm energy of the ginger move the Qi and dispel the Cold and Damp. Grate a 10 cm piece of fresh root ginger and simmer in 4 cups of water for five to ten minutes. Strain off the liquid and keep in a pan. Soak a towel or cloth in the hot liquid and place over the lower back, as hot as you can stand. Cover with a dry towel to keep in the heat. When the cloth begins to cool, put it back into the hot liquid and re-apply; repeat at least three times. Do this three or four times each day to greatly relieve pain and spasm.	• If the pain is severe • If there is numbness, tingling or weakness in the leg • If there are also urinary or bowel symptoms • If symptoms gradually worsen and new symptoms appear
A generally healthy diet (*see page 59*) with the addition of chestnuts and walnuts. You can also eat small amounts of lamb's kidney in soup or chopped into rice porridge (*see page 60*) once weekly.	Do Burnishing laterally on UB23 (*see page 94*), and Kneading or Vibrating on K7, CV4 and K3 (*see pages 91, 95 and 98 for techniques, and pages 26–28 for points*).	Depending upon the energetic pattern, consider *Yao Tong Pian*, *Liu Wei Di Huang Wan* or *Jin Gui Shen Qi Wan*; decide which is most appropriate. You can also use the rubbing oil *Die Da Wan Hua You*. (*See pages 118–125.*)	
	Do Grabbing technique (*see page 93*) on GB21, GB20 and UB10 for neck pain (*see pages 26–28 for points*).	*Xiao Yao Wan* (*see page 124*) if there is associated emotional tension.	

SYMPTOM

Backache (continued)

to the focusing exercises (*see page 51*). You may also consider visualization (*see also page 51*) which will heal the back and strengthen the Kidney energy. The breathing exercise is also beneficial for neck and shoulder tension.

In Chinese medicine there are considered to be two main causes of back pain, plus three other causes for localized pain.

UPPER BACK
Pain here is associated with imbalance in the Heart and Lung. A Lung imbalance may also exhibit symptoms of cough, tiredness, sadness and breathlessness. A Heart imbalance may also show symptoms of palpitations, anxiety and dream-disturbed sleep.

MIDDLE BACK
Pain in this area is associated with an imbalance in the Spleen and Stomach, such as a weakness in the Qi or an obstruction to the flow of Qi in that area. Associated symptoms may be poor appetite, tiredness, abdominal distension, indigestion, loose stools.

Common Cold

The name of this condition reveals the ideas about its cause – cold. Climatic factors are also considered to be the cause of the common cold according to Chinese medicine: emphasis is placed on cold, heat, wind, damp, dryness and summer-heat. Treatments exist to remove these 'temporary guests' from the body.

When a climatic influence such as wind or cold enters the body, the defensive energy tries to prevent further entry and closes the pores. There is then a struggle between the energy of the climatic influence and the energy of the person. The stronger the person's energy, the greater the symptoms.

There will be high fever with no sweating as well as a stiff neck and pain at the back of the head as this is where the climatic influence enters the body. The person will be averse to cold temperature. The Lungs will be affected, with a tickling sensation in the nose and sneezing. The throat will be dry and sore, the head will feel 'stuffed' and there may be a profuse, watery nasal discharge. Symptoms last one to two days. The main aim of treatment here is to open the pores, produce a sweat and so use the person's energy to eject the climatic influence from the body.

If the person does not have such a strong energy, the symptoms tend to descend into the throat (see sore throat on page 146) and the chest (see cough on page 132). Otherwise, tiredness and lethargy may continue yet with little or no fever. Today, the latter is very common as we lead busy lives; our energy becomes depleted and we cannot throw off such climatic factors.

Constipation

This is the passage of faeces every other day or, less frequently, difficulty in passing a hard stool. In long-standing cases there may be lower abdominal discomfort, reduced appetite, belching and headache. In Chinese medicine there are considered to be three causes.

There may be Coldness affecting the Intestines secondary to Kidney Yang weakness. The constipation will be accompanied by chilliness, low back pain, tiredness, frequent urination and vaginal discharge.

There may be Heat affecting the Intestines, leading to dryness of the stools; they will be dry and 'bitty'. There may be associated symptoms of restlessness, agitation, night sweats and thirst.

There may be obstruction to the smooth flow of Liver Qi, leading to an interruption to the normal functioning of the Intestines. There may also be irritability, abdominal distension, belching or flatulence and headache at the side of the head.

TREATMENT

Diet	Massage	Herbs	Seek professional help
	Knead UB13 and UB15 (*see pages 91 and 95*) and do Grabbing (*see page 93*) on GB21 (*see pages 26–28 for points*).		
	Use Vibrating technique on CV12 (*see page 98*), and do Kneading (*see pages 91 and 95*) on St36, UB20 and UB21 (*see pages 26–28 for points*).		
It is important not to overeat during an acute fever otherwise there will be problems later as the food cannot be digested properly and will then generate more heat within the body. This is the origin of the saying, 'Starve a cold or you feed a fever'. Eat a light diet of broths and thin soups. You can also eat soft rice porridge (*see page 60*) with sliced fresh root ginger and spring onion stalk, and fresh steamed vegetables. If there is a fever, eat Chinese cabbage, mung beans, turnips and peas.	Knead Lu7 and LI4, and add LI20 for a blocked nose (*see pages 91 and 95*); do Burnishing on GV16 and UB12 (*see page 94*), do Buffing on Yintang, and add Taiyang for headache (*see pages 90 and 97*); also do Grabbing on GB20 (*see page 93*) for headache. (*See pages 26–28 for points.*)	*Sang Yu Jin* or *Yin Qiao Jie Du Pian* (*see pages 122 and 124*). Drink ginger or sage tea (*see page 117*). The following is also helpful: slice an onion and bring to the boil in 4 cups of water. Simmer for twenty minutes. Add a pinch of cayenne pepper and drink half a cupful, warm, three times daily. Go to bed and sweat out the cold.	• If symptoms persist longer than five days • If symptoms develop in other areas; for example, diarrhoea and vomiting (Stomach involvement) or cough with sputum and breathlessness (Lung involvement) • If there are repeated attacks
A healthy diet (*see page 59*); add walnuts and chestnuts. Avoid cold, raw food. Eat foods of warm energy (*see page 55*). Eat chopped lamb's kidney in soup or in rice porridge (*see page 60*).	Knead K7 and Liv3 (*see pages 91 and 95*), do lateral Burnishing on UB23, UB57 and UB25 (*see page 94*), and do Vibrating on St25, CV6 and CV4 (*see page 98*). (*See pages 26–28 for points.*)	Strengthen Kidney Yang with *Jin Gui Shen Qi Wan* (*see page 120*).	• If symptoms are severe • If there is constipation with bleeding • If symptoms worsen • If it alternates with diarrhoea (constipation one day followed by diarrhoea then next, and so on) • If constipation is associated with vomiting and abdominal bloating
A generally healthy diet (*see page 59*) with the addition of more cooling foods; avoid spices and foods of hot energy (*see page 55*).	Do Kneading (*see pages 91 and 95*) on St25, UB37, LI11 and LI4 (*see pages 26–28 for points*).	*Run Chang Wan* (*see page 122*).	
A generally healthy diet (*see page 59*) with the addition of foods which smooth Liver Qi (*see page 55*).	Knead Liv3, UB25, UB57 and UB37 (*see pages 91 and 95*). (*See pages 26–28 for points.*)	*Xiao Yao Wan* (*see page 124*).	

SYMPTOM

Cough

This indicates that an imbalance is present in the Lungs *(see also page 34)*. In Chinese medicine, the Lung is known as the 'tender organ' as it is the one which is affected by climatic factors. In addition, sadness and loss often manifest as Lung symptoms. For recurrent Lung symptoms such as cough, it is recommended to take up a regular Qi Gong practice, meditation and daily exercise of swimming or walking. Most coughs are mild in nature and are relatively easy to treat yourself; three of the most common types are discussed here.

CHESTY COUGH

This may be caused by invasion of a climatic influence as was discussed in relation to the common cold. The problem here is more severe, as the influence has descended into the Lungs interrupting the normal flow of Qi. This type of situation can occur in people who say 'a cold always goes onto my chest'. The symptoms will be those of the common cold with cough. There may or may not be sputum.

DRY COUGH

Cough may also be caused by internal factors such as Dryness in the Lungs due to lack of fluid (Yin). Smoking and living or working in dry, hot conditions may be a factor; here there will be cough with little or no sputum, dry mouth and perhaps dry skin.

PHLEGMY COUGH

A cough with lots of phlegm is usually due to a weakness of the Lung and the Spleen. Dampness accumulates because of the Spleen weakness and ascends to the Lungs. It collects there causing cough with sputum. Here there is cough with sputum, tiredness, muzzy head, poor appetite and loose stools.

Cystitis

This is a burning sensation when urinating. Associated symptoms may be frequency of urination, frequent desire to urinate, cloudy urine, passing small amounts of urine, pain in the lower abdomen, pain in the lower back and, in severe cases, blood in the urine and fever.

In Chinese medicine this is caused by Heat and Dampness affecting the Urinary Bladder. There is usually some degree of obstruction to the smooth flow of Liver Qi (hence the common association between cystitis and emotional symptoms), Kidney weakness and Spleen weakness.

Depression

The term depression is a loose one which is often applied to a low mood. It may be used to describe sadness, weeping, unhappiness, dissatisfaction and so forth. It is important to try to distinguish the particular quality of the depression in order to determine which organ,

There may be a sense of sadness and loss. This can be experienced after a bereavement or separation and may persist in some people. This is normal and natural, but treatment can help us transform these feelings. In Chinese medicine the Lung is associated with letting go. Symptoms include depression, characterized by sadness, weeping and sighing. There may also be Lung symptoms of pale face, tiredness, cough and, in severe cases, breathlessness.

TREATMENT

Diet	Massage	Herbs	Seek professional help
The diet under common cold is helpful in the first stages. Later, eat foods which strengthen the Lungs (soups, chicken, dates, honey and malt sugar). Add Asiabell root (*Dang Shen*), ginseng (*Ren Shen*) and yellow milk-vetch root (*Huang Qi*). Avoid greasy food, seafood, spicy food, alcohol and tobacco.	Do Kneading on Lu5 and LI4 (*see pages 91 and 95*) and Burnishing on UB13 (*see page 94*). (*See pages 26–28 for points*).	Consider either *Yin Qiao Jie Du Pian* or *Sang Ju Yin* for the acute symptoms. When these have subsided, consider strengthening Lung energy with either *Bu Zhong Yi Qi Wan* or *Liu Jun Zi Wan*. (*See pages 118–125.*) Sage tea is also helpful (*see page 117*).	• If symptoms are persistent – longer than seven to ten days • If there is also breathlessness • If there is coughing with blood
A generally healthy diet (*see page 59*) with the addition of steamed foods to help moisten the Lungs. Avoid greasy food, seafood, spicy food, alcohol and tobacco.	Use Vibrating technique on UB13, Lu9 and K6 (*see page 98*). (*See pages 26–28 for points*).	Consider either *Chuan Bei Pi Pa Gao* or, if chronic, *Yang Yin Qing Fei Tan* (*see pages 118 and 124*).	
A healthy diet (*see page 59*). Avoid cold, raw food; eat warm foods and those with warm energy (*see page 55*). Strengthen the Lungs with soups, chicken, dates, honey and malt sugar. Add 10 g Asiabell root (*Dang Shen*), 5 g ginseng (*Ren Shen*), 10 g yellow milk-vetch root (*Huang Qi*) to vegetable soup (*see page 59*). Avoid or reduce foods which lead to Dampness and eat foods which resolve it (*see page 55*).	Do Kneading on UB20, CV12, St36, UB13 and St40 (*see pages 91 and 95*). (*See pages 26–28 for points*).	When tiredness and poor appetite are less evident, take *Er Chen Wan* in warm climates. When there are signs of tiredness, poor appetite and loose stools take *Liu Jun Zi Wan*. *Chuan Bei Jing Pian* clears white sputum from the Lungs. Use *Chuan Bei Pi Pa Lu* or *Qing Qi Hua Tan Wan* when there is yellow sputum. (*See pages 118–125.*) Also, drink coltsfoot flower tea (*see page 115*).	
A generally healthy diet (*see page 59*) with the avoidance of foods with hot energy (*see page 55*) and greasy and fried food. Eat mung beans, peas, grapes and red beans; also eat rice porridge (*see page 60*) with 30 g purslane. Add salt or white sugar to taste at the end.	Do Stroking and Vibrating on CV3 and UB23 (*see pages 90 and 98*), and Kneading on Sp6, Sp9, Liv5 and K10 (*see pages 91 and 95*). (*See pages 26–28 for points.*)	Consider either *Qian Lie Xian Wan* or *Yu Dai Wan* (*see pages 122 and 124*).	• If symptoms are severe • If symptoms are persistent – longer than three to four days
A generally healthy diet (*see page 59*) with the addition of steamed foods to benefit the Lungs. Also, eat soups, chicken, dates, honey and malt sugar. Add ingredients to vegetable soup as described under phlegmy cough (*see above*).	Do Kneading on Lu7 and P6 (*see pages 91 and 95*), Vibrating on CV17 (*see page 98*), and Pressing on UB13 (*see pages 91 and 96*). (*See pages 26–28 for points.*)	Consider *Bu Zhong Yi Qi Wan* (*see page 118*).	• If symptoms are severe • If depression is accompanied by suicidal thoughts or urges

SYMPTOM

Depression (continued)

in terms of Chinese medicine, is affected. An imbalance of any of the five organs may lead to depression.

Meditation is extremely helpful in dealing with such states of mind. I would very much encourage you to explore the exercises described in chapter three (*see page 51*). Also consider Qi Gong exercises, especially the Fusion of the Five Elements on page 70. Such practices strengthen our minds, calm the Spirit and provide mental and emotional stability. Massage is also important in encouraging emotional states to come to the surface and disperse.

There may be a general feelings of not being able to move forward in your life. There will be what the Chinese refer to as a 'stuckness'. The Liver is associated with the smooth flow of Qi; there will be associated symptoms of anger, irritability, pre-menstrual symptoms of headaches, sore and distended breasts and painful periods, headaches at the side of the head, belching, indigestion and difficulty getting off to sleep at night.

The thoughts and emotions may be overactive and merely 'churn over' — they occupy our mind but do not actually go anywhere. This is to do with the Spleen, which deals with transformation — not just of food but also of mental and emotional states. Depression arising from this organ is to do with 'not moving', an inability to 'digest' thoughts and emotions. There may be associated symptoms of poor appetite, loose stools, nausea and tiredness.

There may be a feeling of unhappiness and a sense of loneliness; there is a general lack of joie de vivre. Associated symptoms include palpitations, insomnia, anxiety and discomfort in the chest. Severe cases may be associated with strong feelings of unworthiness and even suicidal thoughts.

Depression may be more a case of lack of drive and ambition. There may be an apathy, a lack of direction in your life and a feeling that you 'can't be bothered'. In severe cases there may be deep despair. This can alternate with periods of excessive drive and overwork. The Kidneys are associated with the will, and ambition depends upon this organ.

Diarrhoea

This is looseness of the stool, usually several times each day. There are three main situations: the first two are acute cases due to a specific factor, and the third is the chronic form which is long-lasting.

This may be caused by eating cold, greasy or generally unhealthy food. There will be diarrhoea with abdominal pain, rumbling in the abdomen, feelings of cold which are better for warm applications, and no thirst.

This is when the body becomes overheated, as seen in hot climates. There will be diarrhoea which is hot, offensive and yellow, a burning sensation in the anus, dark urine, and in more severe cases there is fever and thirst.

TREATMENT

Diet	Massage	Herbs	Seek professional help
A generally healthy diet (*see page 59*) with the addition of foods which smooth the flow of Liver Qi (*see page 55*).	Knead Liv3, P6 and GB34, and add GB41 for headaches (*see pages 91 and 95*), use Stroking technique on CV12 (*see page 90*), and do Grabbing on GB20 for headaches (*see page 93*). (*See pages 26–28 for points.*) For painful periods and pre-menstrual symptoms see page 144.	*Xiao Yao Wan* (*see page 124*).	
A generally healthy diet (*see page 59*) with no cold or raw food. Eat foods which are warm in energy and those which nourish Qi and Yang (*see page 55*).	Do Pressing on St36 (*see pages 91 and 96*) and Vibrating on CV12 and Sp4 (*see page 98*). (*See pages 26–28 for points.*).	*Bu Zhong Yi Qi Wan* and *Liu Jun Zi Wan* (*see pages 118 and 120*).	
A generally healthy diet (*see page 59*) with the addition of foods to nourish the Blood (*see page 55*).	Use Kneading technique on H7, P6, CV14 and UB15 (*see pages 91 and 95*). (*See pages 26–28 for points.*)	*Gui Pi Wan* (*see page 120*).	
A generally healthy diet (*see page 59*) with the addition of walnuts and chestnuts. You can eat a small amount of sliced lamb's kidney in a soup or rice porridge (*see page 60*) once a week.	Do Burnishing laterally on UB23 (*see page 94*), knead K3 (*see pages 91 and 95*) and do Vibrating on CV4 (*see page 98*). (*See pages 26–28 for points.*)	For weakness of Kidney Yang (Fire) use *Jin Gui Shen Qi Wan*, and for weakness of Kidney Yin (Water) use *Liu Wei Di Huang Wan* (*see page 120*). Refer to each and decide which is best for your situation.	
A generally healthy diet (*see page 59*). Do not eat late at night (after about 7pm), eat regularly and eat warm food.	Do Stroking and Kneading on St25, UB25, St36 with CV12 and CV6 (*see pages 90, 91 and 95*). (*See pages 26–28 for points.*) Applying warmth to the stomach area and lower abdomen helps.	*Ping Wei Pian* or *Xiang Sha Yang Wei Pian* (*see pages 120 and 124*).	• If symptoms are persistent — more than three to four days • If symptoms are severe • If there is diarrhoea with blood • If there is diarrhoea with mucus • If there is diarrhoea in babies and the elderly, because of the risk of dehydration
Eat a light diet avoiding foods of hot energy (*see page 55*). Eat more cooling and cold foods (*see page 55*). Iced drinks are not helpful as they are too extreme and weaken the Qi.	Use Stroking and Kneading techniques on St25, UB25, St36, St44, Sp9 and LI4 (*see pages 90, 91 and 95*). (*See pages 26–28 for points.*)	*Ping Wei Pian* or *Ren Dan* (*see pages 120 and 122*).	

SYMPTOM

Diarrhoea (continued)

There may be weakness of the Spleen and Stomach Qi; associated symptoms include mild abdominal pain, abdominal rumbling, poor appetite, abdominal bloating and tiredness. More severe cases are associated with Coldness in the limbs and 'cock-crow' diarrhoea (at dawn), indicating a weakness of the Kidney Yang; there may be frequent urination and low back pain.

Earache

This is pain or discomfort in the ear. It occurs in babies and children in particular, and can be very distressing. Parents may also be anxious about what it may lead to — fear of mastoiditis, inflammation of the bony area behind the ear, despite the extreme rarity of this condition.

The most frequent cause of earache, according to Chinese medicine, is the accumulation of Dampness (mucus) which rises up from the Stomach and into the Lung. There is also weakness of the Qi of the Spleen and Lung. In Chinese medicine such a picture is known as 'infantile phlegmy'. The main aim of treatment is to strengthen the Qi of the Spleen and Lung as well as resolving Dampness (mucus).

Headaches

There are many different types of headache. They vary widely in their location, severity, duration and quality in individual cases; the most common types are included here. Headaches tend to worry people, so if you are in any way concerned, seek a professional opinion (see also guidelines opposite).

Chinese medicine differentiates headaches according to their location: the three most common locations are given here.

FRONT OF HEAD

These headaches arise from imbalances in the Stomach; this is where 'ice-cream headaches', due to Stomach Cold, are located. They tend to be dull and relieved by eating, particularly warm food. They may come on if a meal is missed or after eating certain foods. There may be associated bowel disturbances or nausea. Treatment is directed at strengthening the Stomach Qi and harmonizing the flow of Qi in the upper digestive tract.

SIDE OF HEAD

These arise from the Liver and Gall Bladder, and are associated with stressful situations which lead to obstruction to the flow of Liver Qi, or with eating certain foods such as shellfish, cheese, chocolate or red wine. If there is an associated Stomach imbalance there may be nausea or vomiting — this is often described as 'Liver Attacking Stomach'. The main aim of treatment is to smooth the flow of Liver Qi and to strengthen the Stomach Qi.

TOP OF HEAD

Headaches here tend to be vague, dull and worse for standing or exercise. They usually come on at the end of the day and are associated with tiredness. They are due to weak Qi and Blood (the Qi and Blood are not sufficient to reach the uppermost parts of the body). The main aim of treatment is to strengthen Qi and Blood. This tends to take some time and rest is very important.

TREATMENT

Diet	Massage	Herbs	Seek professional help
A generally healthy diet (*see page 59*). Do not eat any cold or raw food, and eat more foods of warming energy (*see page 55*). Use fresh root ginger and cinnamon bark in your cooking.	Do Stroking and Vibrating on St25, CV12, UB25, St36, UB20, Liv13 and Sp3 (*see pages 90 and 98*). Add UB23, K3, CV4 and GV20 if there are signs of Kidney involvement. (*See pages 26–28 for points.*)	For Spleen and Stomach Qi weakness use *Xiang Sha Yang Wei Pian* or *Bu Zhong Yi Qi Wan* (stronger). Use *Jin Gui Shen Qi Wan* for Kidney involvement. (*See pages 118–125.*) Drink ginger or fennel tea (*see pages 115 and 117*).	
For long-term health use a generally healthy diet (*see page 59*). You should also refer to the recommendations for diet in babies and infants on page 54; these will go a long way to prevent the development of these problems.	For acute earache Knead SJ5 and GB41 (*see pages 91 and 95*), and do Grabbing on GB20 (*see page 93*). When this has subsided, strengthen the Qi by Kneading St36 and LI4, Stroking CV12 (*see page 90*) and Burnishing laterally on UB20 (*see page 94*). (*See pages 26–28 for points.*)	Drip warmed (care!! not hot) almond or olive oil into the ear. Do not do this if there is discharge from the ear.	• If earache is severe • If there is also high fever • If earache is persistent – longer than two to three days
A generally healthy diet (*see page 59*) with the addition of foods of warm energy as well as those which strengthen Qi and Yang (*see page 55*).	Use Kneading technique on CV12, St36, Sp4 and Yintang (*see pages 91 and 95*). (*See pages 26–28 for points.*)	Drink fennel or ginger tea (*see pages 115 and 117*).	• If headaches are severe • If headaches are progressive • If there is associated vomiting • If there is stiffness of the neck and dislike of light • If there are also symptoms such as weakness of an arm or leg, numbness or tingling • If headaches are gradually worsening
A generally healthy diet (*see page 59*) with the avoidance of foods which are excessively heating (*see page 55*). Smooth the flow of Liver Qi by means of the foods described on page 55.	Strengthen the Stomach by Kneading St36, CV12 and Sp4 (*see pages 91 and 95*). Smooth the flow of Liver Qi by Kneading Liv3, GB34 and P6, and Grabbing GB20 (*see page 93*). (*See pages 26–28 for points.*)	*Xiao Yao Wan* (*see page 124*). You can also apply a cut lemon to the temple, or wash a cabbage leaf, press until the juice begins to leak out, warm the leaf and apply to the painful area.	
A generally healthy diet (*see page 59*) with no raw or cold foods. Eat foods which nourish the Blood and those which strengthen the Qi and Yang (*see page 55*).	Do Burnishing on UB17, UB18 and UB20 (*see page 94*), Stroking and Kneading on CV6 and CV12 (*see pages 90, 91 and 95*), and Kneading on Sp10, Liv3 and St36. (*See pages 26–28 for points.*)	Strengthen the Qi with *Bu Zhong Yi Qi Wan*, and strengthen the Blood with *Dang Gui Pian*. Strengthen the Qi and Blood with *Ba Zhen Wan, Ren Shen Yang Rong Tang* or *Shi Chuan Da Bu Wan*. (*See pages 118–125.*)	

SYMPTOM

Hot Flushes and Menopausal Symptoms

The menopause in women is an important stage in life. In effect, it is a normal event and is only associated with symptoms when there is some imbalance. There are often associated psychological issues which need to be addressed due to changing roles as the children grow up and leave home, and as the relationship with the partner readjusts itself. Meditation practice is of inestimable benefit in allowing us to deal with life changes. It strengthens us and leads to clarity and insight. In this way, the next phase of life will be smoother, healthier and less problematic.

There are many approaches which can benefit women at this time. Commonly, the Kidney energy begins to decline, especially the Yin (Water). As this diminishes, the Kidney and Liver become overheated and lead to symptoms of hot flushes and emotional instability. Heat in the Heart causes sweating, anxiety and insomnia. The main approach of treatment is to support the Kidney and calm the Liver and Heart.

Indigestion

This is discomfort in the upper abdomen in the area of the Stomach. There are three main causes according to Chinese medicine.

Irregular eating tends to injure the Spleen and Stomach. There may be associated symptoms such as distension in the upper abdomen, pain which is worse for pressure, belching with an unpleasant taste in the mouth and a poor appetite. Treatment is aimed at strengthening the Spleen and Stomach and harmonizing the Qi in the upper digestive tract.

There may be an obstruction to Liver Qi attacking the Stomach, where there will be associated symptoms such as nausea, acidity, abdominal distension, irritability and poor appetite. Treatment is aimed at strengthening the Spleen and Stomach as well as smoothing the flow of Liver Qi.

There may be weakness of Stomach Qi with Cold in the Stomach. There will be associated symptoms of cold feelings in the upper abdomen perhaps with frontal headache.

Infantile Colic

This is abdominal pain in infants and young babies. It is more common in babies fed on cow's milk and those who are weaned early. Consider the information on page 54 about a healthy diet for babies and infants.

There may be the ingestion of Cold either from consuming cold food or drink or from contaminated food (food poisoning). Milk and food may obstruct the flow of Qi due to irregular feeding, overfeeding, the consumption of food that is difficult to digest or sleeping immediately after feeding. 'Winding' the baby after food is helpful to prevent this.

TREATMENT

Diet	Massage	Herbs	Seek professional help
A generally healthy diet *(see page 59)*, avoiding foods which are hot in energy *(see page 55)*. Eat walnuts and chestnuts or eat small amounts of sliced lamb's kidney in a soup or rice porridge *(see page 60)* once a week.	Do Vibrating on H7, K3, Sp6 and Liv3 *(see page 98)*, and Burnishing on UB23, UB15 and UB18 *(see page 94)*. For excess sweating massage do Burnishing also on K6 and Lu7. *(See pages 26–28 for points.)*	*Gui Pi Wan (see page 120).*	• If there are severe mental or emotional symptoms
A generally healthy diet *(see page 59)* with an emphasis on warm food and root vegetables.	Knead St36, P6 and St44 *(see pages 91 and 95)*, do Stroking on CV12 *(see page 90)*, and do Buffing on Liv13 *(see pages 90 and 97)*. *(See pages 26–28 for points.)*	*Shen Chu Cha (see page 122).* You can also add a pinch of nutmeg and black pepper to a cup of warmed milk and sip slowly.	• If there is severe pain • If there is abdominal rigidity • If the pain is worse for movement
A generally healthy diet *(see page 59)* with the addition of foods which smooth the flow of Liver Qi *(see page 55)*.	Do Kneading on St36 and P6 with Liv3 and Liv14 *(see pages 91 and 95)*, and Stroking on CV12 *(see page 90)*. *(See pages 26–28 for points.)*	*Shu Gan Wan* or *Xiao Yao Wan (see page 124).*	
A generally healthy diet *(see page 59)* and avoid cold food completely.	Knead St36, P6 and Sp4 *(see pages 91 and 95)*, do Stroking on CV6 and CV12 *(see page 90)*, and Burnishing laterally on UB20 *(see page 94)*. *(See pages 26–28 for points.)*	Drink fennel or ginger tea *(see pages 115 and 117)*. Use *Xiang Sha Yang Wei Pian (see page 124)*. Local warmth from hot water bottles is also helpful.	
This is extremely important in children as they commonly develop digestive disorders. Follow the recommendations for a healthy diet in babies and infants *(see page 54)*.	See treatment routine for Infant Digestive Blockage on pages 100–101.		• If the symptoms are severe

SYMPTOM

Injury

Any injury to the body in the form of a direct blow, a sprain or a strain, leads to obstruction of the flow of Qi and Blood in the local area. The injury causes the Blood to leave the vessels and collect in the tissues, and therefore it cannot flow normally in that area, which leads to an obstruction in the flow of Qi. The resultant symptoms include pain, swelling and bruising. Long-term there may be pain and discomfort with weakness of the affected area. Prompt treatment of the injury will reduce the bruising and pain and lessen the possibility of long-term problems. The quicker that the obstruction to the Qi and Blood can be treated, the sooner the normal healing abilities of the body can begin.

The precise treatment will depend upon the area injured, but massage to the points, compresses, gentle exercise and herbs are helpful in overcoming the effects in the shortest possible time.

Insomnia

There are several ways in which sleeplessness may manifest; four are given here. The exact pattern will give a guide to the underlying energetic imbalance and, consequently, how to address it.

There may be difficulty falling asleep associated with dreams, poor appetite, general tiredness, palpitations and waking in the night. The mind cannot settle and churns thought over and over. This is weakness of the Blood and Spleen Qi.

There may be waking in the night with low back pain, dizziness, tinnitus, urinary symptoms (frequent urination, urination at night, dribbling urination) and irritability. This is due to an imbalance between the Heart and Kidney.

There may be depression, anger, headaches, especially at the sides of the head, pain in the upper abdomen at the side, a bitter taste in the mouth and dreams which disturb the sleep. This is due to Fire in the Liver.

Sleeplessness may be associated with indigestion, distension of the abdomen and belching. This is due to an imbalance in the Stomach.

TREATMENT

Diet	Massage	Herbs	Seek professional help
Eat a generally healthy diet (*see page 59*), and avoid cold and raw food.	The points vary according to the site injured (*see pages 26–28 for points*). When Qi and Blood are obstructed points become tender: these are known in Chinese as *Ah Shi* points and are discussed under backache. *Neck:* SI3, UB10, GB21; *Shoulder:* GB21, LI15, SJ14, LI14; *Elbow:* LI11, LI10, LI12, LI4; *Wrist:* SJ4, SJ5; *Hip:* GB30, GB29, GB34; *Knee:* Xiyan, St44, Sp9, GB34; *Ankle:* St41, GB40, UB60. Do Kneading or Grabbing as appropriate (*see pages 91–96*). Massage joints with vinegar (*see page 89*) to relieve stiffness and relax tendons.	Older people should use *Du Huo Ji Sheng Wan* (*see page 120*). Use the rubbing oil *Die Da Wan Hua You* (*see page 118*). For the initial stages after the injury use a seaweed compress to cool the inflammation. Place a small amount of kelp in a pan with 4 cups of water. Bring to the boil and simmer for twenty minutes. Soak a piece of gauze or lint in the liquid when cool, and bandage to the affected area. Use sage tea (*see page 117*) or chrysanthemum flower infusion (*see page 115*) if bruising is present.	• If there is severe pain • If the injury is accompanied by shock (sweating, pallor, rapid and thready pulse) • If there is inability to move a joint • If there is marked swelling and bruising
A generally healthy diet (*see page 59*) with the addition of foods which nourish the Blood and those with warming energy (*see page 55*), particularly root vegetables. Avoid tea and coffee.	Knead UB20 and UB15 (*see pages 91 and 95*) and Nip-knead (using the thumbnail – *see page 101*) H7, P6 and Sp6. Do Vibrating on Yintang and Anmian (*see page 98*).(*See pages 26–28 for points.*)	*Ding Xin Wan* or *Gui Pi Wan* (*see pages 118 and 120*). Also, drink 1 tablespoon of blackstrap molasses (this is unrefined) in a glass of warmed milk before bed.	• If associated with severe mental or emotional symptoms
A generally healthy diet (*see page 59*).	Nip-knead points as above, Knead UB15, UB23 and K3 (*see pages 91 and 95*), and do Vibrating on points as above. (*See pages 26–28 for points.*)	Consider *Liu Wei Di Huang Wan* (*see page 120*).	
A generally healthy diet (*see page 59*) with foods which smooth the Liver Qi (*see page 55*). Avoid foods of hot energy (*see page 55*).	Knead H7, P6, Sp6 with GB12, GB34 and Liv2 (*see pages 91 and 95*), do Burnishing laterally on UB18 and UB19 (*see page 94*), and Vibrating as above. (*See pages 26–28 for points.*) Rubdown is also helpful (*see page 93*).	*Xiao Yao Wan* (*see page 124*).	
A generally healthy diet (*see page 59*). Do not eat after 7pm. Avoid cold and raw food, and eat regularly. Eat foods of warm energy (*see page 55*) with plenty of root vegetables.	Do Kneading on H7, P6, Sp6 with UB21 and St36 (*see pages 91 and 95*), do Stroking on CV12 (*see page 90*), and do Vibrating as above (*see pages 26–28 for points.*)	*Liu Jun Zi Wan* (*see page 120*). Also, drink 1 tablespoon of blackstrap molasses (this is unrefined) in a glass of warmed milk before bed.	

SYMPTOM

Nasal Blockage, Nasal Discharge

These symptoms are centred around the head and nose, and are due to the collection of mucus in that area. The nose may be blocked or there may be nasal discharge which is white or, in more severe cases, yellow or green. Frontal headache is common. The symptoms can be severe with extreme pain in some cases, particularly if the mucus is thick and does not move. The sinuses will be tender to the touch, and there may be a feeling of 'muzziness' in the head, especially in the mornings.

There may be weak Lung Qi, weak Spleen Qi and Damp (mucus) accumulation which collects in the sinuses. In energetic terms, this is a relatively minor condition as the Qi is strong enough to hold the imbalance in the nose, rather than it descending into the Lungs themselves. There may be associated symptoms of tiredness, poor appetite, loose stools, desire for sweet foods and indigestion.

There may be Fire in the Liver and Gall Bladder which ascends to the head. There may be associated symptoms of irritability, headaches, pain at the sides of the body, belching and hot feelings in the head.

Nausea and Vomiting

These are essentially the same symptom – nausea is merely the milder form. The Stomach Qi normally descends; if it ascends this is experienced as nausea or vomiting. In Chinese medicine there are four situations that may lead to these symptoms.

Motion sickness is caused by a pre-existing imbalance in the Spleen and Stomach, often with Damp accumulation in the Stomach. Treatment aims to strengthen both organs and resolve Dampness so that the Qi descends and flows more harmoniously.

There may be irregular eating, particularly of rich, fatty or cold food. There will be indigestion (see this specific symptom), belching, poor appetite, constipation and offensive wind.

There may be obstruction to the smooth flow of Liver Qi which then 'attacks' the Stomach, causing belching, pain in the upper abdomen at the sides, irritability or anger and acid regurgitation.

There may be weakness of Spleen and Stomach Qi. Associated symptoms will be poor appetite, loose stools, tiredness, and discomfort or nausea after eating a large meal.

Numbness and Tingling

This is common, especially in women and those engaged in repetitive actions of one part of the body. Symptoms may vary in severity. There may be mild tingling which can develop into shooting pains. Eventually there may be weakness of the muscles; numbness can occur later.

In terms of Chinese medicine the cause of these symptoms is obstruction to the flow of Qi and Blood in the channels of the affected area. There may be an associated accumulation of Dampness, which would indicate a Spleen imbalance also. In addition, there is frequently weakness of Blood, which then tends to flow less smoothly. Repetitive activity will place a greater strain on the Qi and Blood flowing in the channels.

TREATMENT

Diet	Massage	Herbs	Seek professional help
A healthy diet (*see page 59*) with steamed foods to benefit the Lungs; add soups, chicken, dates, honey and malt sugar. Add 10 g Asiabell root (*Dang Shen*), 10 g white atractylodes (*Bai Zhu*) and 6 g Chinese yam (*Shan Yao*) or ingredients as for phlegmy cough (*see page 133*) to vegetable soup. Eat warm foods and those which resolve Dampness; avoid foods which generate it (*see page 55*).	Use Kneading technique on Lu5, Lu9, CV12, St36, Sp3, LI20 and LI4 (*see pages 91 and 95*). (See pages 26–28 for points.)	*Bi Yan Pian* (*see page 118*). Use *Liu Jun Zi Wan* (*see page 120*) long-term after the acute episode has subsided to strengthen Lung and Spleen Qi and to transform Dampness (mucus). *Er Chen Wan* (*see page 120*) is for Damp (mucus) accumulation in a person with generally strong energy.	• If there is nasal discharge after head injury
A generally healthy diet (*see page 59*) with the addition of foods which smooth the flow of Liver Qi (*see page 55*). Avoid those foods of hot energy (*see page 55*).	Knead Liv3, GB34, LI20, LI4 and CV12 (*see pages 91 and 95*). Use Grabbing technique on GB20 (*see page 93*). (*See pages 26–28 for points.*)		
A light diet of warm, nourishing food before travelling. Avoid greasy, heavy, excessively sweet and cold food.	Knead P6 (see pages 91 and 95) and do Stroking on CV12 (*see page 90*). (See pages 26–28 for points.)	*Ren Dan* (*see page 122*). A warm tea made from fresh root ginger (*see page 117*) to sip whilst travelling is also useful.	• If there is thirst, dark and scanty urine, dry mouth; such dehydration is more likely in babies and the elderly and is also seen earlier • If nausea and vomiting are not relieved by your self-help strategy • If symptoms are accompanied by weight loss • If there is vomiting with blood • If symptoms are caused by food eaten several days before
Eat a healthy diet (*see page 59*) to avoid such symptoms. During an attack, eat light, warming food.	Do Kneading on St36, CV12, P6, Sp4 with St25 (*see pages 91 and 95*). (*See pages 26–28 for points.*)	*Shen Chu Cha* and *Xiang Sha Yang Wei Pian* (*see pages 122 and 124*).	
A generally healthy diet (*see page 59*) with the addition of foods to smooth the flow of Liver Qi (*see page 55*).	Do Kneading on St36, P6, Sp4 with Liv3 (*see pages 91 and 95*), and Stroking on CV12 (*see page 90*). (*See pages 26–28 for points.*)	*Shu Gan Wan* or *Xiao Yao Wan* (*see page 124*).	
A generally healthy diet (*see page 59*) with the addition of foods which are warm in energy and those which strengthen the Qi and Yang (*see page 55*).	Do Pressing on UB20 (*see pages 91 and 96*), Stroking as above, and Kneading on St36, P6 and Sp4 (*see pages 91 and 95*). (*See pages 26–28 for points.*)	*Bu Zhong Yi Qi Wan* or *Liu Jun Zi Wan* (*see pages 118 and 120*).	
A generally healthy diet (*see page 59*) with the addition of warming foods and those which strengthen Qi and Yang, as well as foods to strengthen Blood (*see page 55*).	Knead St36, Sp10, H7 and Liv3 (*see pages 91 and 95*), do Stroking on CV12 (*see page 90*), and Burnishing laterally on UB17 and UB18 (*see page 94*). (*See pages 26–28 for points.*)	There are several patents of help here. The best ones to begin with are those which strengthen Qi and nourish Blood. *Ba Zhen Tang* and *Shi Quan Da Bu Tang* help both. *Dang Gui Pian* is a good Blood tonic. (*See pages 118–125.*)	• If symptoms are severe • If there is also weakness or paralysis

SYMPTOM

Pain and Stiffness in Joints and Muscles

These symptoms are due to obstruction to the flow of Qi and Blood in the channels. The obstruction may be caused by various factors, but the common ones are climatic: wind, cold and damp. There will be a preceding weakness in Qi or Blood, or both, which allows such climatic influences to enter the body.

There will be pain in the joints with stiffness, numbness and swelling. In severe cases there may even be deformity of the joints. Wind manifests as 'wandering' pains. Dampness is characterized by heaviness, stiffness and swelling. Cold causes joints and affected areas to be painful and feel cold to the touch; warmth relieves the symptoms. In some people, the invading climatic factor may turn into heat. Here there will be redness, swelling and heat in the affected area; this may correspond to rheumatoid arthritis. Treatment is more complex in such cases and you may need to seek professional help.

Painful Periods

This is an extremely common symptom which is often easily remedied by Chinese medicine. The important question to ask is when the period becomes painful: is it at the beginning of the period, or later on? These are the two main categories that are recognized.

Some women develop pain just before the period starts and it lasts for the first one or two days of the period. The pain tends to be cramping in nature and there may be clotty menstrual blood which is perhaps purplish or dark. This is caused by obstruction to the smooth flow of Liver Qi. There may be associated symptoms of irritability, headaches and sore and distended breasts. In some women there may be a degree of Cold in the uterus. Severe cases may be associated with fainting, diarrhoea and headaches. Avoid cold drinks and foods such as ice-cream during menstruation.

Some women develop pain later in the period. It tends to be dull and dragging in nature. There may be associated symptoms of tiredness, dull headaches, anxiety, insomnia and feeling cold, and the period may be heavy. This is due to Blood deficiency, usually associated with weakness of the Liver and Kidney.

Pre-menstrual Symptoms

These are common in our modern society. The menstrual cycle is an interesting example of a cycle of nature, and this is something that Chinese medicine understands very well. Women often feel very different mentally and emotionally at different times of their cycle. In traditional cultures, the women would withdraw from society at the time of the period and this would be an opportunity to engage in more spiritual or artistic pursuits (this may not be so easy now in our modern society!). However, if women can begin to become aware of these changes they can start to change their lifestyle. Merely doing this may relieve symptoms of pre-menstrual syndrome.

There may be some degree of Spleen Qi weakness leading to tiredness, desire for sweet food and fluid retention.

TREATMENT

Diet	Massage	Herbs	Seek professional help
A generally healthy diet *(see page 59)* with the addition of foods which nourish the Blood *(see page 55)*, particularly celery and parsley. Also eat foods of warming energy and those which strengthen Qi and Yang *(see page 55)*.	Do Rubdown on Sp21 for generalized aches and pains *(see page 93)*. Specific points are as follows *(see pages 26–28 for points)*: *Shoulder:* LI15, LI14, SJ14, SI9, SI10 *(and see Rowing on page 92)*; *Elbow:* LI10, LI11, LI12; *Wrist:* SJ4, LI5, SJ5; *Hip:* GB30, GB29, UB37; *Knee:* St34.; Xiyan, GB34, Sp9; *Ankle:* St41, UB60, K3. Do Kneading or Grabbing as appropriate *(see pages 91–96)*.	*Du Huo Ji Sheng Wan (see page 120)*. You can also drink 2 teaspoons of apple cider vinegar and honey in warm water three times daily.	• If symptoms are severe • If symptoms are worsening
A generally healthy diet *(see page 59)*, avoiding cold and raw food.	Do Vibrating on CV6 and CV3 *(see page 98)*, and Kneading on Liv 3, Sp10 and GB34 *(see pages 91 and 95)*. *(See pages 26–28 for points.)*	*Xiao Yao Wan (see page 124)*. Drink warm cinnamon tea *(see page 115)* to warm the uterus and lower abdomen. Hot water bottles to the lower abdomen may also help; the Qi flows more smoothly if it is warmed.	• If symptoms are severe • If there is very heavy menstrual bleeding
A generally healthy diet *(see page 59)* with the addition of foods to nourish the Blood and Yin and those of warm energy *(see page 55)* and plenty of root vegetables.	Do Burnishing and Kneading on UB17, UB18 and UB23 *(see pages 91–95)*, Kneading on K3 and Liv8, and Vibrating on CV4 *(see page 98)*. *(See pages 26–28 for points.)*	*Gui Pi Wan, Ba Zhen Wan, Ren Shen Yang Rong Wan* and *Dang Gui Pian* all help nourish the Blood *(see pages 118–125)*. Determine which is most appropriate for your situation.	
A generally healthy diet *(see page 59)* with the addition of warming foods and those which strengthen Qi and Yang *(see page 55)*.	Do Stroking on CV12 *(see page 90)* and Knead St36, Sp4 and UB20 *(see pages 91 and 95)*. *(See pages 26–28 for points.)*	*Bu Zhong Yi Qi Wan (see page 118)*; symptoms of obstruction to the smooth flow of Liver Qi as described below may be worsened by this formula as the energy becomes stronger. If there are mixed symptoms of Spleen Qi weakness and obstruction to the smooth flow of Liver Qi, add *Xiao Yao Wan (see page 124)* before your period also.	• If the symptoms are severe.

SYMPTOM

Pre-menstrual Symptoms (*continued*)

Stagnation of Liver Qi leads to irritability, sensitivity, sore breasts, headaches and a general feeling of tension. There may be lower abdominal pain just before the period begins and also for the first few days of the period.

Sore Throat

This symptom is much more common in children than adults. The throat may be sore or, in severe cases, painful. There may be fever and an associated difficulty in swallowing. The lymph glands in the neck will be swollen and tender. The tonsils themselves may be enlarged and red, with white or yellow discharge on their surface. The tongue will have a thickish yellow coat and the person will feel generally ill. In Chinese medicine, there are two causes of such symptoms.

Enlarged tonsils with discharge are due to Heat in the Stomach or Lungs which flares up into the throat when there is an acute invasion of WindCold or WindHeat. If symptoms recur, consider professional treatment to eradicate the underlying tendency.

Some people get recurrent attacks of sore throat which are not associated with enlargement of the tonsils or a yellow or white discharge on them. If it is a mild symptom, it is almost certainly not tonsillitis but due to Kidney or Liver energy which flares up to the throat and causes mild discomfort, dryness, soreness and redness. There may also be tiredness and low backache.

Sputum

This is the production of mucus from the Lungs. It is frequently associated with cold and damp climates. In severe cases it may be associated with breathlessness. Smoking and dusty atmospheres tend to make it worse.

In Chinese medicine this condition is considered to be caused by an accumulation of Dampness in the Lungs due to a weakness in Lung and Spleen energy. The Spleen produces Dampness because it cannot transform food efficiently and this Dampness rises up to collect in the Lungs. The main aim of treatment is to strengthen the Spleen and Lungs and to transform the accumulation of Dampness.

Vaginal Discharge

This is a common symptom and may be associated with fungal infections such as 'thrush' (Candida). There are two main types of discharge that are included here: white and yellow.

WHITE
There is usually some degree of Spleen Qi weakness with an accumulation of Dampness (mucus) which sinks down into the lower abdomen. This may also collect in the Intestines. Associated symptoms will be desire for sweet food, poor or disturbed appetite, tiredness, swelling due to water retention and loose stools. There may be a weakness of Kidney Yang in addition.

YELLOW
There may be obstruction to the smooth flow of Liver Qi. The discharge will be yellowish as Heat is often generated as a result of this obstruction to flow. Associated symptoms are pre-menstrual breast soreness, headaches at the sides of the head, irritability, discomfort at the sides of the abdomen, belching and bowel disturbances (constipation or irregular consistency of the faeces).

TREATMENT

Diet	Massage	Herbs	Seek professional help
A generally healthy diet *(see page 59)* with the addition of foods which smooth the flow of Liver Qi *(see page 55)*.	Do Kneading on Liv3, GB34 and Liv14 *(see pages 91 and 95)* and use Buffing technique on UB18 *(see page 90)*.	*Xiao Yao Wan (see page 124)*.	
A light diet during an attack of sore throat is helpful. Avoid foods which are hot in energy and eat more foods which are cooling *(see page 55)*.	Use Kneading technique on Lu10, LI4, St44 and SJ17 *(see pages 91 and 95)*. *(See pages 26–28 for points.)*	*Sang Ju Yin* or *Yin Qiao Jie Du Pian (see pages 122 and 124)*. Also, use sage gargle *(see page 117)*.	• If there is pain in the throat (rather than soreness).
A generally healthy diet *(see page 59)* with the addition walnuts and chestnuts. You can also eat small amounts of sliced lamb's kidneys in soup or rice porridge *(see page 60)* once weekly.	Knead K3, K6, Lu10 and Lu7 *(see pages 91 and 95)*. *(See pages 26–28 for points.)*	Consider *Liu Wei Di Huang Wan (see page 120)*.	
A generally healthy diet *(see page 59)* with those foods which help transform Dampness; reduce or avoid those foods which generate Dampness *(see page 55)*.	Do Kneading on St36, Sp3, St40 and Lu5 *(see pages 91 and 95)* and Vibrating on CV12 *(see page 98)*. *(See page 26–28 for points.)*	*Chuan Bei Jing Pian* for cough with white sputum, and *Chuan Bei Pi Pa Lu* or *Qing Qi Hua Tan Wan* for cough with yellow sputum. Use *Liu Jun Zi Wan* if there are also symptoms of Spleen Qi deficiency. *(See pages 118–125.)* Coltsfoot flower tea is also helpful *(see page 115)*.	• If you are feverish • If there is green sputum • If there is breathlessness • If there is blood in the sputum
A generally healthy diet *(see page 59)* with foods which resolve Dampness *(see page 55)*. Avoid or reduce foods which generate Dampness and eat foods of warm energy *(see page 55)*.	Do Stroking and Vibrating on CV6 and CV12, and add CV4 for low backache and tiredness *(see pages 90 and 98)*. Knead Sp6, St36, Sp9 and UB23, and add K7 for low backache and tiredness *(see pages 91 and 95)*. *(See pages 26–28 for points.)*	A specific formula for Damp accumulation is *Er Chen Wan*. *Jin Gui Shen Qi Wan* strengthens the Kidney Yang, and *Liu Jun Zi Wan* strengthens the Spleen Qi and transforms Dampness. *(See pages 118–125.)* Use these when acute symptoms of itching and soreness have subsided.	• If there is red or bloody discharge • If there is black, green or offensive discharge
A generally healthy diet *(see page 59)*; add foods which smooth the flow of Liver Qi and those which resolve Dampness *(see page 55)*. Eat rice porridge *(see page 60)* with the addition of purslane, and avoid foods of hot energy and those which generate Dampness *(see page 55)*.	Do Stroking and Vibrating on CV6, CV12 and CV3 *(see pages 90 and 98)*, and Kneading on Sp6, St36, Sp9, UB23, Liv5 and K10 *(see pages 91 and 95)*. *(See pages 26–28 for points.)*	*Yu Dai Wan (see page 124)*.	

CHAPTER EIGHT

PRACTITIONERS
TECHNIQUES AND TRAINING

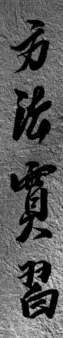

- *Choosing a practitioner*
- *What to expect at a consultation*
- *Methods of diagnosis and professional techniques*
- *Training in Chinese medicine*

This chapter offers guidance on choosing a practitioner of Chinese medicine with whom you can feel comfortable and confident, as well as discussing the techniques they may use in their practice. Professional methods of diagnosis are also introduced, and for those who may be interested in training in Chinese medicine, there is advice on how to select a college or school that offers professional training.

HOW TO CHOOSE A PRACTITIONER

There are several levels on which you may seek treatment from a professional. I know from my own practice that each person has their own reason. There may be a specific symptom causing you discomfort or limitation; there may be a general feeling that 'things are not right' without there being a particular symptom or disease; or you may wish to receive treatment to maintain a good level of health and so prevent problems developing later (increasingly the case as Chinese medicine becomes more widely known).

Seeking help from a health practitioner is an important decision, especially if the method of treatment is not one with which you are familiar. It is generally advisable to seek help from a registered practitioner; however, different countries have different regulations concerning registration, and some practitioners choose, for a variety of reasons, not to be registered. They may be experienced and professional people, so you will need some sort of system to check on individual practitioners. The following criteria are particularly useful to consider when you make your evaluation.

TRAINING

It is essential that you consider the practitioner's training; where did they train and how long did they train for? There is a bewildering array of qualifications and certificates in Chinese medicine: checking directly with the practitioner is the best way to find out what they mean. Details of national regulations and accredited organizations can be found on page 157.

LANGUAGE BARRIERS

It is also important to find out whether there are any language or cultural barriers between yourself and the practitioner. If there are, it may not necessarily present a problem; there may be a translator in the clinic and the practitioner may be skilled in pulse, tongue and observation methods of diagnosis of Chinese medicine (*see page 151 for further discussion*). However, if you wish to discuss personal issues this may not be possible if the practitioner has limited skill in your language. This aspect is more to do with personal preference, since it will depend on the individual as to what situation they feel more comfortable with.

ATMOSPHERE OF TREATMENT

Treatment is not just about formal qualifications and training. It is also about how you feel with this particular person. Healing takes place in an atmosphere of relaxation, with feelings of trust and security; this means that your personal connection with the practitioner (and theirs with you) is the single most important thing to consider. Remember that you may be discussing personal feelings and thoughts, and you will certainly be experiencing a treatment which can affect you quite deeply. It is far more effective, and certainly more curative, when you feel comfortable with the practitioner.

GETTING INVOLVED

I would encourage you to be actively involved in your health programme, so discuss this with your practitioner. Ask lots of questions, but also take their recommendations. In this way, you will reap the benefits of the treatment more quickly and fully.

Before you begin treatment, find out how long the treatment will last and how often you will need to see the practitioner. It is best to discuss these aspects right at the start, so that you know exactly what to expect as your treatment progresses.

COST

The price of a treatment is dependent on many factors; the location of the clinic is the main consideration. For example, an appointment will cost much more in New York City than in rural Ireland. Price is certainly something that you should check out – try to find out the going rate in your area. Discuss it with your practitioner before attending so that you are clear about how much treatment will cost (it is usual to pay extra for herbs).

CHECK-LIST

These are the most important issues to consider when choosing a practitioner:

- *Check on the practitioner's training.*
- *Try to see someone who has been personally recommended by a friend or another practitioner who you know.*
- *Discuss your case (including fees) with the practitioner before finally deciding upon treatment.*

A VISIT TO A PROFESSIONAL

All medical practitioners have a particular way of obtaining information with which to make a diagnosis and then begin treatment. Chinese medicine has its own specific methods of diagnosis, of which pulse and tongue diagnosis are skilled arts. This section guides you through what happens on your first visit to see a practitioner of Chinese medicine.

CONSULTATION

The exact format of the consultation will depend upon each individual practitioner. Generally, appointments tend to be fairly long – at least half an hour, and in some cases up to an hour. In this time, a case history will be taken, symptoms noted and information gathered about current levels of health as well as past medical history. The tongue and pulse will be examined and a diagnosis in terms of Chinese medicine made on the basis of this information.

There are three main ways in which a diagnosis is made: listening to the symptoms (which indicate the nature and location of the imbalance), feeling the pulse and looking at the tongue. Pulse and tongue diagnosis are discussed below.

Pulse diagnosis

The pulse is felt at the wrist, and this gives information about the energies within the body and their relative balance. In Chinese medicine, pulse diagnosis is a refined art and it takes many years to become an expert. Traditionally, masters of pulse diagnosis are able to tell you of events in your childhood that have led to current problems.

The pulse on each side of the wrist is different, and there are three positions on each side relating to different organs (see illustration right). The right side is to do with Qi and gives information about Lung, Spleen and Kidney Yang. The left side is to do with Blood and gives information about Heart, Liver and Kidney Yin.

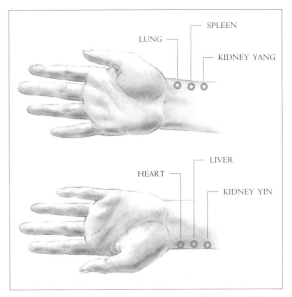

Assessing the pulse at specific positions on the wrist enables a professional practitioner to diagnose where the imbalance is likely to be within the body.

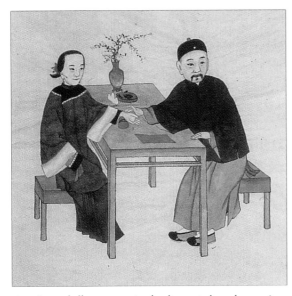

A traditional illustration of pulse diagnosis by a doctor of Chinese medicine. This nineteenth-century watercolour is from 'Chinese Trades and Professions' by Zhou Pei Qun.

At each position, the practitioner considers the energy, the pulse rate and the quality of the energy. For example: a wiry pulse feels like a taut wire, indicating a Liver imbalance; a slippery pulse feels like 'rolling pearls on a jade plate' and indicates the presence of Dampness or Phlegm within the body; and a choppy pulse feels like 'scraping a sharp knife along a piece of bamboo' and indicates weakness of Blood. There are many other pulse qualities that can be deduced, and the information from the pulse gives the practitioner a good idea of the imbalance and where it is within the body.

Tongue diagnosis

The tongue contains information about the whole body (as is the case with all organs); reflexology and iridology are based upon the same idea. Different organs are represented in different areas on the tongue (see overleaf).

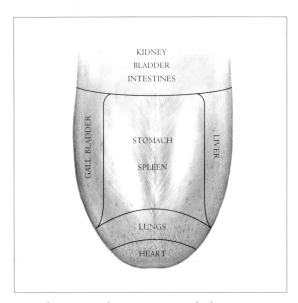

Particular areas on the tongue represent the different organs of the body. This allows the practitioner to examine the tongue and make a diagnosis accordingly.

The colour of the tongue indicates the amount of Qi in the body: a pale tongue means weakness of Qi or Blood, or both; a red tongue indicates Heat within the body; and a red centre to the tongue means that there is Heat in the Stomach. The condition of the tongue also gives information about different organs. For example, a tongue with teethmarks along the edge indicates weak Spleen Qi, whereas cracks in the tongue usually means that there is Heat drying the fluids in much the same way that hot weather causes cracks to appear in the ground.

The tongue coat indicates the presence of factors inside the body, such as Dampness or an invading climatic factor: a white coat means Cold and a yellow coat means Heat. For example, people with cystitis (*see page 132*) have Dampness and Heat in the Urinary Bladder. They will have a yellow tongue coat present at the back of the tongue.

What happens next

Following on from the diagnosis, a treatment plan and general management strategy will be formulated, which your practitioner will discuss with you. You will learn how you can take an active part in treatment yourself. There may be specific advice about diet, relaxation, exercises, and so forth. Treatment will be given depending upon the practitioner you are consulting and their method of treatment; herbs, massage and acupuncture may be used, as well as advice about diet and exercise.

How to prepare for treatment

There are several recommendations which most practitioners would advise a patient to follow before attending for treatment. As Chinese medicine deals with observation, it is particularly important not to mask any signs or symptoms. Follow the guidelines given below on what to do, or *not* do, before visiting a practitioner.

BEFORE TREATMENT

• *Do not clean or brush your tongue, as this may change the important clinical information determined by tongue diagnosis.*

• *Do not wear strong perfumes or deodorants which may mask important clues.*

• *Avoid alcohol on the day of treatment, especially if you are having acupuncture; there can be unusual adverse reactions.*

• *Do not drink coffee before the consultation as this may change the pulse.*

• *Try to be relaxed if you can, and quietly confident that you are taking the first step towards regaining — and maintaining — your health.*

PROFESSIONAL TECHNIQUES

By now you will know that Chinese medicine incorporates a variety of methods of treatment. The professional methods discussed here are acupuncture, moxibustion and cupping, plus prescribed herbal medicine.

ACUPUNCTURE

This is where fine needles are used to pierce the skin at specific points. The use of a needle, and various manipulations to it, strengthens and balances the Qi. Acupuncture needling is generally painless. Once the needle is inserted, Qi starts to 'arrive' at the needle. The same sensation, known as *De Qi*, is obtained during massage *(see page 91)*. In China, people use a wide variety of terms to describe the sensation: aching, fullness and tingling are but a few. People trained in the Japanese tradition of acupuncture use very shallow needle insertion with much finer needles, and so this sensation is not experienced so much, if at all.

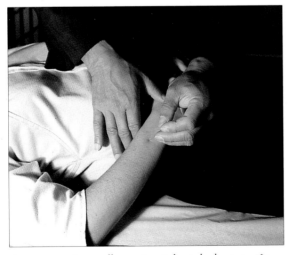

Acupuncture: fine needles are inserted painlessly at specific points to balance Qi and Blood in the body. The sensation experienced – De Qi – indicates that Qi is present.

Length of treatment

The needles are left in place for about fifteen minutes, but this can vary depending on the practitioner and the particular problem being treated. In general, the longer the needles are left in, the stronger the treatment. For people with weaker Qi, practitioners tend to use few needles and also reduce the time for which they are actually inserted in the body.

After treatment

Make sure you do not undertake strenuous exercise or drink alcohol after treatment. Allow the treatment time to give you maximum benefit. Relaxation, a light meal and gentle exercise are fine later that day.

How often?

The frequency of treatments will depend upon the practitioner, their style of acupuncture and the patient's energy. In China, chronic conditions are treated on alternate days; acute problems receive daily treatments (this is not always possible in the West).

When I see someone for the first time, I usually use acupuncture and prescribe a herbal formula; I then see them again some two to three weeks later. After this, in most cases I will see them once a month, with the patient continuing the herbal treatment between visits. For more acute problems, severe disease or where patients need greater support, I see them more often. However, you will need to discuss your particular pattern of treatment with your practitioner when you first attend.

Responses to treatment

There may be various responses: the energy has, to some extent, been rebalanced so there may be feelings of being 'spaced out', tired, energized or just 'different'. These feelings can last for a variable amount of time, but tend to be less noticeable with subsequent treatments as the Qi becomes stronger and more balanced.

Several things may happen to specific symptoms you are having treated. After the first treatment they may actually become stronger for a short time – a few hours or even a day. This is because the treatment has strengthened the energy; it indicates that improvement will follow. This reaction is seen in the healthiest people. Subsequent treatments do not usually produce this reaction.

Some people notice that their symptoms merely start to improve. This, again, is a good response and subsequent treatments will build upon this. Others, and certainly those who have had problems for some time, notice that their specific symptoms may not change for several treatments. This is because the energy imbalance is more fixed. You may, however, feel better 'in yourself': your energy is stronger, you sleep better and you feel generally more comfortable. After some more treatments

your symptoms should begin to improve. This will happen more quickly:

- If they are more recent in origin.
- If you have stronger Qi.
- If you make lifestyle changes and involve yourself in the process of treatment.
- If several things are done at once, such as acupuncture with herbs, exercise and relaxation.

MOXA

Moxibustion, the burning of moxa (a dried herb, mugwort), is a good example of warming treatment. Moxa has warming and energizing properties, and is used on specific points to increase energy and relieve pain.

Moxibustion can be applied in a variety of ways according to the condition. For instance, burning moxa on a slice of ginger enhances the warming quality: the heat of the moxa passes through the ginger into the point being treated. Burning moxa on a needle directs warming energy straight into the point; a moxa stick gives heat to the point over which it is used; and a moxa box applies heat to a large area, helpful for low backache and period pain.

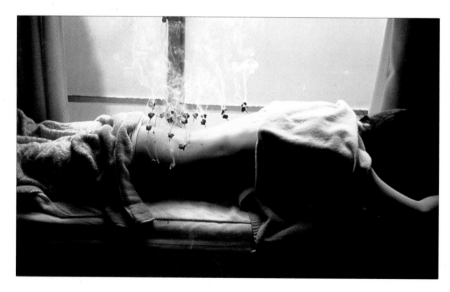

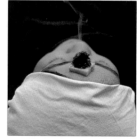

Above. *A cone of moxa is placed on a slice of ginger on the point and then lighted.*

Left. *Burning moxa on needles directs warming energy straight into points.*

CUPPING

This is the application of glass or, traditionally, bamboo cups to specific areas of the body. The cups aid the flow of Qi and Blood in painful conditions, or dispel Wind and Cold in acute conditions, such as colds or fevers.

Before the cup is placed on to the area to be treated, a lighted ball of cotton wool soaked in spirit (or similar) is introduced into the cup for a few moments and then withdrawn. The resultant vacuum allows the cup to stay on the skin; it remains in place for a few minutes (*see right*). Superficial bruising sometimes occurs due to the pressure exerted by the action of the vacuum: this only lasts a few days and is of no consequence unless it is visible (the bruising is not painful).

HERBS

There are hundreds of herbs and patents that are strong in their action and these can only be safely prescribed by a professional practitioner. Herbal consultations tend to be relatively short, perhaps fifteen to thirty minutes long, as only a history and examination is necessary. Most patients are seen again after about two weeks to check on their progress; thereafter, monthly visits are the norm. Always

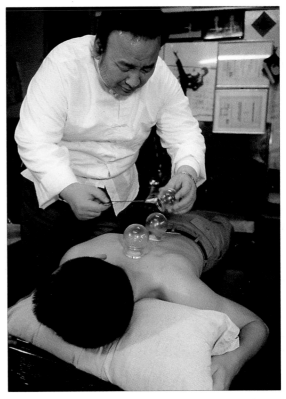

Before the advent of antibiotics, 'cuppers' were employed in hospitals to reduce fever, since cupping dispels Wind and Heat.

report any new symptoms or apparent adverse reactions to your practitioner immediately – do not wait for the next appointment.

TRAINING IN CHINESE MEDICINE

Practising Chinese medicine is a highly rewarding occupation. It is an opportunity to help others and to develop your own inner healing potential. If you are interested in training in Chinese medicine yourself, there are certain aspects you should consider.

ACCREDITATION OF COLLEGES

Increasing numbers of people are attending colleges and schools of Chinese medicine to train in this form of healing. There are many different colleges of differing traditions, which reflects the diversity of Chinese medicine and its spread from the East. Some schools are excellent and offer professional training at a high level. It is helpful to check a school's history, what type of training is on offer and, more importantly, where the training leads. For instance, is registration and accreditation possible after qualification?

COST

Training in Chinese medicine is a financial load and there may not be grants or public funds available to help you. Most people who train in Chinese medicine tend to be in their mid twenties to mid fifties, and so already have another occupation. You may find that you have to work at the same time as studying, which will place a greater strain on your time and energy; it is also likely to affect your family as well, so bear this in mind.

CLINICAL TRAINING

I trained in acupuncture in China, as have many acupuncturists and herbalists. One of the attractions is the sheer number of people attending clinics – I saw more patients in a day than attend some Western clinics in a week! Whole hospitals in China are devoted to the practice of Chinese medicine, and this richness of clinical experience is invaluable when treating your own patients. Obviously, training in China is not a feasible option for most people, so the best thing you can do is make sure that the school clinic where students train is busy, so you are exposed to many different situations in a safe, supervised way.

TREATMENT STYLES

There are many ways of applying the principles of Chinese medicine; there is no one right way to do so and it is helpful for students to be aware of the range available. For instance, there are different influences from countries such as Japan, Vietnam and Korea; the Japanese style of acupuncture is described on page 153, and Japanese herbal medicine uses much lower doses of herbs than its Chinese counterpart. However, if too many different styles are taught it can be confusing, so a balance has to be attained. It is better to learn one method thoroughly than many methods superficially.

STUDY

Training in Chinese medicine is hard work and there is a lot to study. However, Chinese medicine is an art, and the *application* of knowledge also has to be given attention. Does the course allow for self-development, the acquisition of counselling skills, the practice of Tai Chi Chuan, Qi Gong and meditation? When you qualify as a professional, you will be discussing such things with your patients. It is essential that you are familiar with them and that they are integrated into your own life.

A GOOD PRACTITIONER

Conventional Western thought compartmentalizes events and thoughts. In reality, patients and practitioners are both interconnected and interdependent. If we, as practitioners, wish to help heal our patients, we need to use these methods in our own lives. Practitioners who do not do so, tend not to be of so much help to their patients. The intention here is not to create a perfect person who imparts their wisdom to others. It is merely a recognition that we all have a tendency to an imbalance of Qi and Blood and need to live according to the principles of Chinese medicine if we wish to be healthy.

The essence of good practice is not so much *what* is done, but rather *how* it is done. This is the practical application of the skills developed by the practice of meditation and Qi Gong; it is a way of 'being' rather than a way of 'doing'. When we, as practitioners or as patients, are able to enter into such a state, true healing occurs and suffering is eased.

RESOURCES

UK

NATIONAL REGULATIONS

At present, no governmental legislation controlling the practice of Chinese medicine. The British Acupuncture Accreditation Board, formed in 1989, guides schools through an accreditation procedure. The Board is an independent organization which lays down minimum standards of training. There is currently one acupuncture register: the British Acupuncture Council. Members are bound by a code of ethics and practice and are fully insured, and may use the letters MBAcA after their names. The minimum training period is three years.

GENERAL ORGANIZATIONS

British Acupuncture Council
Park House
206–208 Latimer Road
London W10 6RE
Tel: 0181 964 0222
(Contact for details of schools and colleges of Chinese medicine.)
Council for Complementary and Alternative Medicine
38 Mount Pleasant
London WC1X 0AP
Register of Chinese Herbal Medicine
21 Warbreck Road
London W12 8NS
(Contact for details of qualified herbal practitioners.)

Register of Chinese Massage Therapy
PO Box 8739
London N28

QI GONG

Linda Chase Broda
The Village Hall
163 Palatine Road
Manchester M20 2GH
Tel: 0161 445 1568
Fax: 0161 445 9568
Zhi-Xing and Zhen-Di Wang
Chinese Heritage
15 Dawson Place
London W2 4TH
Tel/Fax: 0171 229 7187
Lin Jun Wen
3 New College Parade
Finchley Road
London NW3 5EP
Tel: 0171 722 9808
Fax: 0171 722 7341

CHINESE MASSAGE

Sarah Pritchard
196 Wricklemarsh Road
Blackheath
London SE3 8DP
Tel: 0181 856 8757
Julia Clark
3b Bowater Place
Blackheath
London SE3 8ST
Tel: 0181 293 3089
Li Hi
75 Gloucester Road
London SW7 4SS
Tel: 0171 244 9550

HERBAL SUPPLIERS

East—West Herb Shop
3 Neal's Yard
London WC2H 9DP
Harmony Ltd
627 High Road
Leytonstone
London E11 4PA
Mayway
43 Waterside Trading Estate
Trumper's Way
Hanwell
London W7
Number One Herb Company
36 Bankhurst Road
London SE6 4XN

AUSTRALIA

NATIONAL REGULATIONS

There is currently no state registration of acupuncturists. There is some movement towards this but at the moment the situation is similar to the UK. The main organization is the Australian Acupuncture Association which represents about seventy-five per cent of Chinese medicine practitioners. They are bound by a professional code of ethics laid down by the Association.

GENERAL ORGANIZATIONS

Acupuncture Ethics and Standards Organization
PO Box 84
Merrylands
NSW 2160

Australian Acupuncture Association
PO Box 5142
West End
Brisbane 4101

QI GONG

Jack Lim
The Qi gong Association of Australia
458 White Horse Road
Surrey Hills
Victoria 3127
Tel: 03 9836 6961
Fax: 03 9830 5608
Allan Kelson
Chi Kung Institute
GPO Box 66
Adelaide 5001
Tel/Fax: 08 828 74422

CHINESE MASSAGE

David Freeland
6–15 Raine Street
Bondi Junction
NSW 2022
Tel: 02 524 4620
Tel: 02 387 2982

HERBAL SUPPLIERS

Chinese and Herbal Centre
1st Floor
392–394 Sussex Street
Sydney
NSW 2000
Chinese Ginseng Herb Co.
75–77 Ultimo Road
Haymarket
NSW 2000

FURTHER READING

Bensoussan, Alan, *The Vital Meridian.* Edinburgh: Churchill Livingstone, 1991.

Craze, Richard, *Feng Shui for Beginners.* London: Hodder and Stoughton, 1994.

Craze, Richard and Tang, Stephen, *Chinese Herbal Medicine.* London: Piatkus, 1995.

Fratkin, Jake, *Chinese Herbal Patent Formulas.* Boulder, CA: Shya Publications, 1986.

Jilin, Liu (ed.) *Chinese Dietary Therapy.* Edinburgh: Churchill Livingstone, 1995

Kohn, Livia (ed.), *Taoist Meditation and Longevity Techniques.* University of Michigan Press, 1989.

Kwok, Man-Ho with O'Brien, Joanne, *The Elements of Feng Shui.* Dorset: Element, 1991.

Maciocia, Giovanni, *The Foundations of Chinese Medicine.* Edinburgh: Churchill Livingstone, 1991.

MacRitchie, James, *Chi Kung: Cultivating Personal Energy.* Dorset: Element, 1993.

Mitchell, Stephen (trans.), *Tao Te Ching* (Lao-Tzu). London: Kyle Cathie Ltd, 1990.

Ni, Maoshing (trans.), *The Yellow Emperor's Classic of Medicine (Neijing SuWen).* Boston, MA: Shambhala, 1995.

Reid, Daniel, *Chinese Herbal Medicine.* Boston, MA: Shambhala, 1987.

Reid, Daniel, *The Tao of Health, Sex and Longevity.* London: Simon & Schuster, 1989.

Rinpoche, Sogyal, *The Tibetan Book of Living and Dying.* London: Rider, 1992.

Teeguarden, Ron, *Chinese Tonic Herbs.* Tokyo: Japan Publishers, 1984.

Unschuld, Paul, *Medicine in China.* Los Angeles, CA: University of California Press, 1985.

Van Alphen, Jan and Aris, Anthony (eds.), *Oriental Medicine.* London: Serindia Publications, 1995.

Wiseman, Nigel, Ellis, Andrew, and Zmiewski, Paul, *The Fundamentals of Chinese Medicine.* Brookline, MA: Paradigm Publications, 1985.

Zhu, Chun-Han, *Clinical Handbook of Chinese Prepared Medicines.* Brookline, MA: Paradigm Publications 1989.

INDEX

THE AUTHOR AND THE CONSULTANTS

Dr Stephen Gascoigne M.B., Ch.B, C.Ac., Dip.CHM qualified in medicine at Liverpool University in 1976. He worked as a general practitioner before opening his own practice in nutrition and allergy testing in 1983. In 1985 he trained in acupuncture at the Shanghai International College of Chinese Medicine and he went on to open his own acupuncture practice, which he runs today near his home in West Cork, Eire. He qualified in Chinese herbal medicine at the London Academy of Oriental Medicine in 1993, and is author of *Prescribed Drugs and the Alternative Practitioner,* and *The Manual of Conventional Medicine for Alternative Practitioners.* The latter has become the set textbook for many colleges of alternative medicine both in the UK and the US. He lectures at a number of colleges, including the Integrated College of Chinese Medicine in Reading, England.

James MacRitchie Dipl.Ac.(NCCA), B.Ac.(UK) is a teacher and widely acclaimed author on Qigong (*Chi Kung: Cultivating Personal Energy,* Element Books 1993, and *The Chi Kung Way: Alive with Energy,* Harper-Collins 1997), and publishes 'The International Chi Kung/Qigong Directory' (available from the address below). He has been practising Classical Acupuncture since 1977, co-directs The Chi Kung School at The Body-Energy Center, and is a Council Member of The World Academic Society of Medical Qigong (Beijing, China). He is Founding President of The Chi Kung/Qigong Association of America.
He can be contacted at:
The Chi Kung School at
The Body-Energy Center
PO Box 19708
Boulder, CO 80308, USA
Tel: 303 442 3131
Fax: 303 442 3141

Robert Cran MA, Dip.CHM & Ac (Nanjing) trained in specialized areas of Chinese medicine at the Nanjing College of Traditional Chinese Medicine, including Chinese massage, acupuncture and specialist herbal departments. He is a member of several professional associations, including the British Acupuncture Council, the Register of Chinese Herbal Medicine and the Register of Chinese Massage Therapy, and in 1991 he founded the London School of Chinese Massage Therapy. He runs his own Chinese medicine practice in London, Durban and Kerala, India.
He can be contacted at:
The Chinese Medicine Practice
253 East End Road
East Finchley
London N2 8AY
Tel/Fax: 0181 444 0103
E-mail address:
101340.1114@compuserve.com

ACKNOWLEDGEMENTS

I am particularly grateful to my teachers, including Nguyen Tinh Thong, who have taught me so much and to my patients who continue to inspire me through their open-heartedness.

There are many people who have helped this book reach completion including, but not only: Lei Zhou An, Ian Breakspear, Stefan Chmelik, Hilary Gascoigne, Angela and John Hicks of the College of Integrated Chinese Medicine, Kirk G. Haney, Stephen Janz, Efrem Korngold, Susan Mears, Alan Treharne, and last but not least Zoë Hughes, Tessa Monina and Pritty Ramjee of Eddison Sadd for their hard work and professional expertise. Special thanks also to Robert Cran and Jim MacRitchie for their valued contributions.

PICTURE CREDITS

12 (bronze figure) Reproduced from *Chinese Herbal Medicine,* by Daniel Reid. © 1996 Kümmerly+Frey; 12 Courtesy of The Needham Research Institute; 20 E.T. Archive; 25 Wellcome Institute Library, London; 45 Mountain View, 17th Century Ming Dynasty/ Bridgeman Art Library, London; 46 Keith Cardwell/Impact; 64, 104 Courtesy of The Needham Research Institute; 106 Melanie Friend/The Hutchison Library; 110 J. Hatt/ The Hutchison Library; 151 Wellcome Institute Library, London; 153 Images Colour Library; 154 Agiajara/Visions/Impact; 155 ©1996 Nik Wheeler.

EDDISON SADD would like to thank the following models: Sarah Adie, Robert Cran, Maxine Deslandes, Jacqueline McLellan, Sarah Pritchard, Emma Smith, Lin Jun Wen and Ethan West.

EDDISON•SADD EDITIONS

Project Editor...............................Zoë Hughes
Editor...Tessa Monina
Proofreader..................................Dorothy Frame
Indexer...Pat Pierce

Art Director...........................Elaine Partington
Art Editor.......................................Pritty Ramjee
Photographer.................................Gill Orsman
Make-up Artist...........................Karen Fielding
Still-life photographer........Stephen Marwood
Illustrator...................................Julie Carpenter
Line Artist.....................................Anthony Duke
Picture Researcher........................Liz Eddison

Production............................Hazel Kirkman
                                               Charles James